Bodybuilding Meal Pr

The Ultimate Guide for the Busy Competitive Athlete with 100+ Simple Recipes for Muscle Growth & Mass Gain + Bonuses: 30-Day Meal Plan & Smart Grocery Shopping Tactics

Colton Jones

© Copyright 2023. Colton Jones. - All rights reserved.

The content contained within this book may not be reproduced, duplicated or transmitted without direct written permission from the author or the publisher.

Under no circumstances will any blame or legal responsibility be held against the publisher, or author, for any damages, reparation, or monetary loss due to the information contained within this book. Either directly or indirectly.

Legal Notice:

This book is copyright protected. This book is only for personal use. You cannot amend, distribute, sell, use, quote or paraphrase any part, or the content within this book, without the consent of the author or publisher.

Disclaimer Notice:

Please note the information contained within this document is for educational and entertainment purposes only. All effort has been executed to present accurate, up to date, and reliable, complete information. No warranties of any kind are declared or implied. Readers acknowledge that the author is not engaging in the rendering of legal, financial, medical or professional advice. The content within this book has been derived from various sources. Please consult a licensed professional before attempting any techniques outlined in this book.

By reading this document, the reader agrees that under no circumstances is the author responsible for any losses, direct or indirect, which are incurred as a result of the use of information contained within this document, including, but not limited to, — errors, omissions, or inaccuracies.

Table of Contents

1. **Introduction** 5
   - 1.1 Purpose of the Book 5
   - 1.2 Brief Overview of Bodybuilding Nutrition 7
   - 1.3 Importance of Meal Prep in Bodybuilding 8

2. **Setting the Foundation** 9
   - 2.1 Understanding Macronutrients 9
   - 2.2 Importance of Micronutrients 10
   - 2.3 Hydration and its Role in Muscle Building 11
   - 2.4 Setting Nutritional Goals 12

3. **Getting Started with Meal Prep** 13
   - 3.1 Basics of Meal Preparation 13
   - 3.2 Essential Kitchen Equipment for Efficient Meal Preparation 15
   - 3.3 Grocery Shopping Essentials 17
   - 3.4 Time Management and Scheduling 18

4. **Sunrise Fuel for Your Day** 19

5. **Satisfying Lunchtime Delights to Recharge** 35

6. **Nutrient-Dense Suppers** 61

7. **Smart Snack Choices** 87

8. **Post-Workout Refueling Recipes** 99

9. **Vegetarian and Vegan Delights** 116

10. **Advanced Meal Prep Strategies** 129
    - 10.1 Batch Cooking and Freezing: A Lifesaver for the Busy Bodybuilder 129
    - 10.2 Optimizing Meal Timing: Synchronizing Nutrition with Your Body's Clock 130

11. **Overcoming Challenges** 131
    - 11.1 Balancing Desires: Managing Cravings and Cheat Days 131

11.2 The Journey of Persistence: Staying Motivated and Consistent 132

11.3 Embarking on a Transformative Journey: Encouragement and Final Thoughts 133

12 Bonuses 134

12.1 My 30-Day Meal Plan 134

12.2 Smart Grocery Shopping Tactics 141

12.3 Colton Jones Sample Weekly Grocery list 142

13 Alphabetical Recipe Index 143

1 Introduction

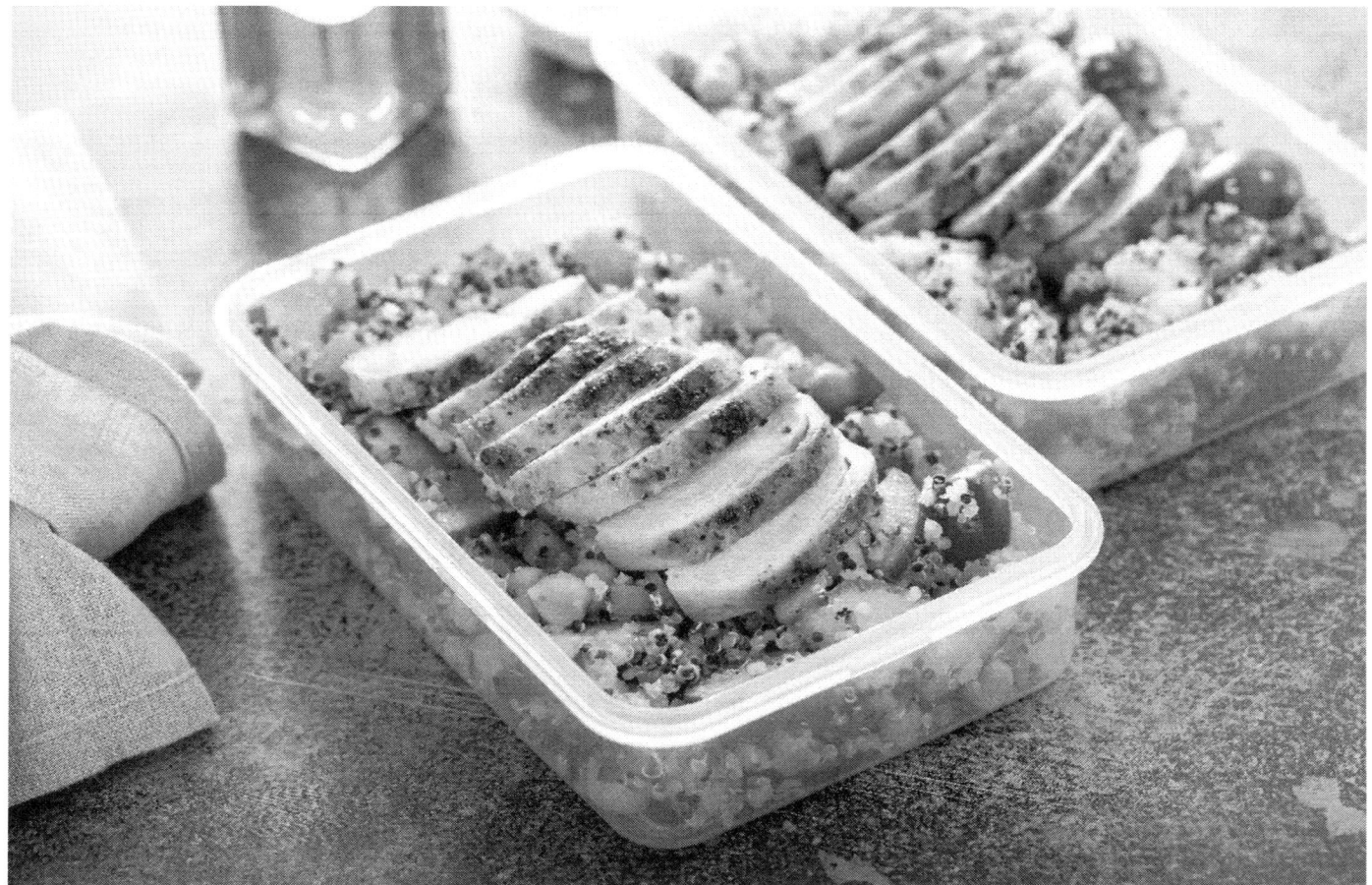

Classic Grilled Chicken Quinoa Tabbouleh - Page 52

1.1 Purpose of the Book

The purpose of this book, intricately woven into its pages, is to serve as a comprehensive guide for those venturing into the world of bodybuilding, eager to integrate optimal nutrition to maximize their gains, a purpose that is multifaceted, aiming not just to educate but also to inspire and empower every individual who seeks to transform their body and enhance their life through disciplined training and mindful eating. It's meticulously crafted to provide profound insights into the science of bodybuilding and the pivotal role of nutrition in building muscle and improving overall health, demystifying the complexities of nutritional science and offering clear, concise, and actionable knowledge on macronutrients, micronutrients, calorie intake, and meal timing, enabling readers to make informed and effective decisions regarding their diet. Beyond the realm of nutritional science, this book emerges as a culinary treasure trove, offering a diverse array of delicious and nutritious recipes specifically designed to cater to the unique dietary needs of bodybuilders, celebrating culinary creativity where flavor meets nutrition, and providing readers with the inspiration and means to explore and enjoy a rich variety of meals that fuel their bodybuilding journey.

Moreover, the purpose extends to inspiring and empowering readers to take control of their nutrition and their body, fostering a sense of self-discipline, commitment, and a passion for healthy living and bodybuilding, instilling a mindset of resilience and determination, enabling individuals to overcome challenges, stay motivated, and relentlessly pursue their bodybuilding and fitness goals. This book adopts a holistic approach to bodybuilding and nutrition, emphasizing the importance of mental well-being, adequate rest, and a balanced lifestyle in conjunction with training and diet, promoting a harmonious integration of all aspects of life to achieve a state of physical and mental equilibrium, thereby enhancing the overall quality of life. Recognizing the uniqueness of each individual, it provides personalized guidance, offering tailored advice, meal plans, and nutritional strategies to accommodate different body types, preferences, and goals, facilitating a personalized journey that allows each reader to discover and embrace their path to bodybuilding success and nutritional well-being.

Furthermore, the book aims to cultivate a sense of community and mutual support among readers, encouraging the sharing of experiences, knowledge, and advice, creating a supportive environment where individuals can connect, learn, and grow together, fostering a collective pursuit of bodybuilding and nutritional excellence. In essence, this book is a beacon of light in your bodybuilding journey, illuminating the path to muscular development and nutritional wisdom, providing you with the tools, knowledge, and inspiration to sculpt your body, nourish your mind, and elevate your spirit, acting as a companion in your quest for physical transformation and a guide in your exploration of the enriching world of nutrition and culinary artistry. Let this book be the catalyst for your transformation, inspiring you to embrace the discipline of bodybuilding, the joy of nutritious eating, and the fulfillment of achieving your dreams, empowering you to transcend limitations, pursue excellence, and experience the profound joy of a healthy, strong, and vibrant life.

1.2 Brief Overview of Bodybuilding Nutrition

Embarking on a bodybuilding journey necessitates a profound understanding of nutrition, serving as the cornerstone for the monumental task of sculpting one's physique. This journey is about more than just lifting weights; it's a delicate balance of consuming the right amount and types of nutrients to fuel muscle growth, enhance performance, and expedite recovery. Whether your goal is muscle gain, or overall performance enhancement, applying the principles of bodybuilding nutrition is pivotal. In this realm, macronutrients stand as foundational pillars. Proteins, sourced from lean meats, dairy, eggs, and legumes, act as the essential building blocks for muscle repair and growth. Carbohydrates, prioritized from whole grains, fruits, and vegetables, serve as the primary energy source, crucial for fueling workouts and aiding in recovery. Fats, obtained from sources like avocados, nuts, seeds, and oils, play a critical role in hormone production, including key hormones like testosterone that are vital for muscle growth.

However, the importance of micronutrients and hydration should not be understated. Despite being required in smaller amounts, vitamins and minerals are crucial for various physiological functions, including metabolism, bone health, and immune function. Adequate hydration is paramount, given water's role in nearly every biochemical reaction within the body. Mastering energy balance is also fundamental; a caloric surplus facilitates muscle gain, while a deficit is essential for fat loss, necessitating a delicate balance to prevent excessive fat gain or muscle loss during respective bulking or cutting phases. The strategy of nutrient timing, which involves consuming the right nutrients at optimal times, can significantly impact recovery and growth, with regular, balanced meals and snacks ensuring a consistent supply of energy and nutrients.

Supplementation, while not a replacement for a well-rounded diet, can offer convenience and fill nutritional gaps. Recognizing that each bodybuilder is unique, the journey requires personalized nutritional strategies, necessitating regular monitoring and adjustments to align with evolving goals, needs, and bodily responses. Moreover, bodybuilding nutrition transcends mere dietary intake; it's interwoven with lifestyle, sleep patterns, stress levels, and overall well-being.

1.3 Importance of Meal Prep in Bodybuilding

Meal prep transcends being merely a practical approach to nutrition; it's a strategic asset with profound implications for your bodybuilding journey, fostering an environment where your nutritional practices are in perfect harmony with your goals, lifestyle, and preferences. This proactive approach is instrumental in ensuring that every morsel you consume propels you closer to your bodybuilding aspirations. It's a system that instills a discipline unparalleled, embedding consistency in your dietary regime. With meals thoughtfully prepared in advance, you eradicate the unpredictability that often accompanies daily nutrition choices, thereby adhering to a regimented, reliable eating plan imperative for bodybuilding success.

Moreover, in the whirlwind of modern life, carving out moments to prepare wholesome meals can be a Herculean task. Herein lies the beauty of meal prep: it's a time-saving grace that bestows the convenience of having nourishing meals at your fingertips, circumventing the allure of nutritionally-void, expedient food substitutes. It's a methodology that affords you meticulous command over portion sizes and caloric intake, a critical component for effective energy balance management, pivotal in all stages, be it bulking, cutting, or maintaining. It guarantees that each prepped meal is a bastion of nutritional equilibrium, delivering the perfect consortium of macronutrients, micronutrients, and fiber, essential for sustained vigor, muscular development, and holistic health.

Meal prep strategy extends its influence to recovery and performance; with post-exercise meals prepped, your body is assured immediate delivery of crucial nutrients, accelerating recovery, spurring muscle protein synthesis, restoring glycogen, and mitigating muscle tenderness, culminating in enhanced athletic performance. This foresight in nutrition also serves as a psychological boon, endowing you with mental tranquility and a sense of empowerment, diminishing food-related stressors, and liberating your focus for training and life's other pursuits. Ultimately, meal prep is the compass that ensures your daily nutritional practices are in unwavering alignment with your overarching bodybuilding ambitions, serving as a tangible testament to your dedication and continually fuelling your journey forward.

2 Setting the Foundation

2.1 Understanding Macronutrients

Understanding macronutrients is foundational for bodybuilders, guiding informed dietary choices, goal-specific nutrition plans, and an optimized bodybuilding path. This knowledge sets the stage for enduring success and peak physical performance. Proteins, the building blocks of life, are indispensable for muscle repair and growth, composed of amino acids essential for muscle protein synthesis, recovery, and maintaining lean mass during weight loss, with sources like lean meats and legumes. Carbohydrates, the body's energy powerhouses, drive workouts and post-exercise recovery. Complex ones from whole grains offer sustained energy, while simple carbs are perfect for post-workout boosts.

Fats, essential for hormone production and overall health, support muscle growth and nutrient absorption, with avocados and nuts being ideal sources. Balancing these macronutrients is crucial; a well-rounded diet optimizes body composition and performance, requiring a tailored approach based on individual goals and metabolism. Timing also plays a role; consuming proteins and carbs around workouts enhances muscle growth and recovery. Personalization is key, as each bodybuilder has unique nutritional needs. Customized plans, considering individual metabolic rates and goals, ensure better adherence and success. Lastly, the quality of macronutrients is vital. Opting for nutrient-dense, whole foods over processed options promotes health, performance, and longevity, providing essential vitamins and antioxidants.

2.2 Importance of Micronutrients

While macronutrients are central to a bodybuilder's diet, micronutrients fine-tune the body's functioning, facilitating muscle growth, recovery, and health. These tiny components, though required in minimal amounts, have a colossal impact, including vitamins, minerals, and specific compounds essential for numerous physiological processes. Minerals like magnesium and calcium are crucial for muscle functions, while vitamins like E and C, acting as antioxidants, mitigate workout-induced muscle damage, expediting recovery. B-vitamins, pivotal in metabolizing macronutrients into cellular energy, directly influence workout intensity and endurance.

Equally vital, minerals such as calcium and vitamin D underpin bone health, a critical aspect for bodybuilders to support increasing muscle mass and the rigors of weightlifting. In the realm of immunity, vitamins like C and A, along with zinc, fortify the immune system, a crucial defense especially as intense training can render athletes prone to illnesses. Additionally, iron's role in oxygen transport is indispensable during workouts for energy production, with deficiencies manifesting as fatigue or reduced endurance. Beyond these, micronutrients are integral to hormonal balance, with elements like zinc and vitamin D involved in producing key hormones, including testosterone and growth hormone.

However, the quest for optimal macronutrient ratios often overshadows the significance of micronutrients, with many bodybuilders inadvertently neglecting micronutrient-rich foods, leading to potential deficiencies. The remedy is dietary diversity. A spectrum of colorful fruits, vegetables, nuts, seeds, lean meats, dairy, and whole grains ensures a rich intake of essential vitamins and minerals. Foods like leafy greens and citrus fruits are abundant in crucial elements like iron, calcium, and vitamin C, while nuts and seeds are excellent sources of magnesium and zinc. Embracing a varied diet is not just about muscle building; it's about nurturing a body capable of extraordinary feats.

2.3 Hydration and its Role in Muscle Building

Hydration, integral to muscle building and athletic prowess, permeates every facet of muscle functionality, growth, and recuperation. Proper hydration strategies not only bolster workout efficacy but also expedite muscle development and thwart injuries, laying the groundwork for triumphant bodybuilding pursuits. This book delves into hydration's intricacies, offering actionable guidance for seamlessly incorporating optimal hydration into your regimen, empowering your quest for muscular augmentation with energy and resilience.

Water, the crux of cellular mechanics, including those in muscle cells, is indispensable for the molecular processes underpinning muscle repair and expansion. It's pivotal in ferrying nutrients, oxygen, and hormones to muscle tissues, while expelling metabolic debris, a process essential for robust energy synthesis, protein construction, and muscular well-being. During strenuous exercise, hydration plays a defensive role, dispersing internal heat and facilitating perspiration, thereby averting thermal stress, sustaining endurance, and forestalling premature weariness.

Moreover, water serves as the principal element of synovial fluid, diminishing joint friction and ensuring their longevity, a critical aspect for seamless, painless mobility fundamental to weightlifting and bodybuilding. However, inadequate hydration can precipitate a downturn in strength, endurance, and muscle responsiveness, culminating in subpar training sessions and hindered muscular advancements. Thus, maintaining optimal water levels is paramount.

Bodybuilders should adhere to steadfast hydration practices: consistent daily water consumption, with guidelines suggesting a minimum of 3 liters for men and 2.2 liters for women, supplemented by additional intake pre, post, and during workouts. Prioritizing pre-workout hydration fortifies water levels, while intermittent sipping during sessions wards off dehydration, and post-exercise rehydration rejuvenates and restores fluid equilibrium. Integrating electrolytes, lost in sweat, is vital to preserve fluid harmony and avert muscular spasms, achievable through electrolyte-infused drinks or nourishments.

2.4 Setting Nutritional Goals

Setting nutritional goals is intrinsic to your bodybuilding journey, serving not just as a guide but as a strategic compass, steering your dietary habits towards a synergy of muscle growth and athletic prowess. These goals, clear and realistic, are the bedrock upon which your bodybuilding ambitions are solidly built, ensuring every morsel you consume is a step towards your ultimate physique. They are the roadmap that navigates you through the complexities of bodybuilding, keeping you focused and ensuring that your nutrient intake, body composition, and performance are optimized.

It's crucial to start with specific goals, whether aiming for muscle mass, fat loss, or enhanced recovery, and these should be realistic, meshing seamlessly with your lifestyle and preferences, avoiding the pitfall of ambition tipping into the unattainable and unsustainable. Your nutritional strategies must echo your training, with strength goals demanding increased protein and calories, while leaning out calls for meticulous calorie and macronutrient management. Constant monitoring and adaptability are key, using feedback from your body and performance to tweak your approach.

Amidst this, never lose sight of the importance of a varied diet; it's not just about meeting macronutrient goals but also ensuring a rainbow of foods on your plate to meet all micronutrient needs. Enlisting professional guidance can be invaluable, providing tailored advice and insights into perfecting your food choices, supplement needs, and portion sizes. And throughout this journey, remember to prioritize protein for muscle repair, manage your energy balance, stay hydrated, and synchronize your meals with your workout routines for peak performance and recovery.

3 Getting Started with Meal Prep

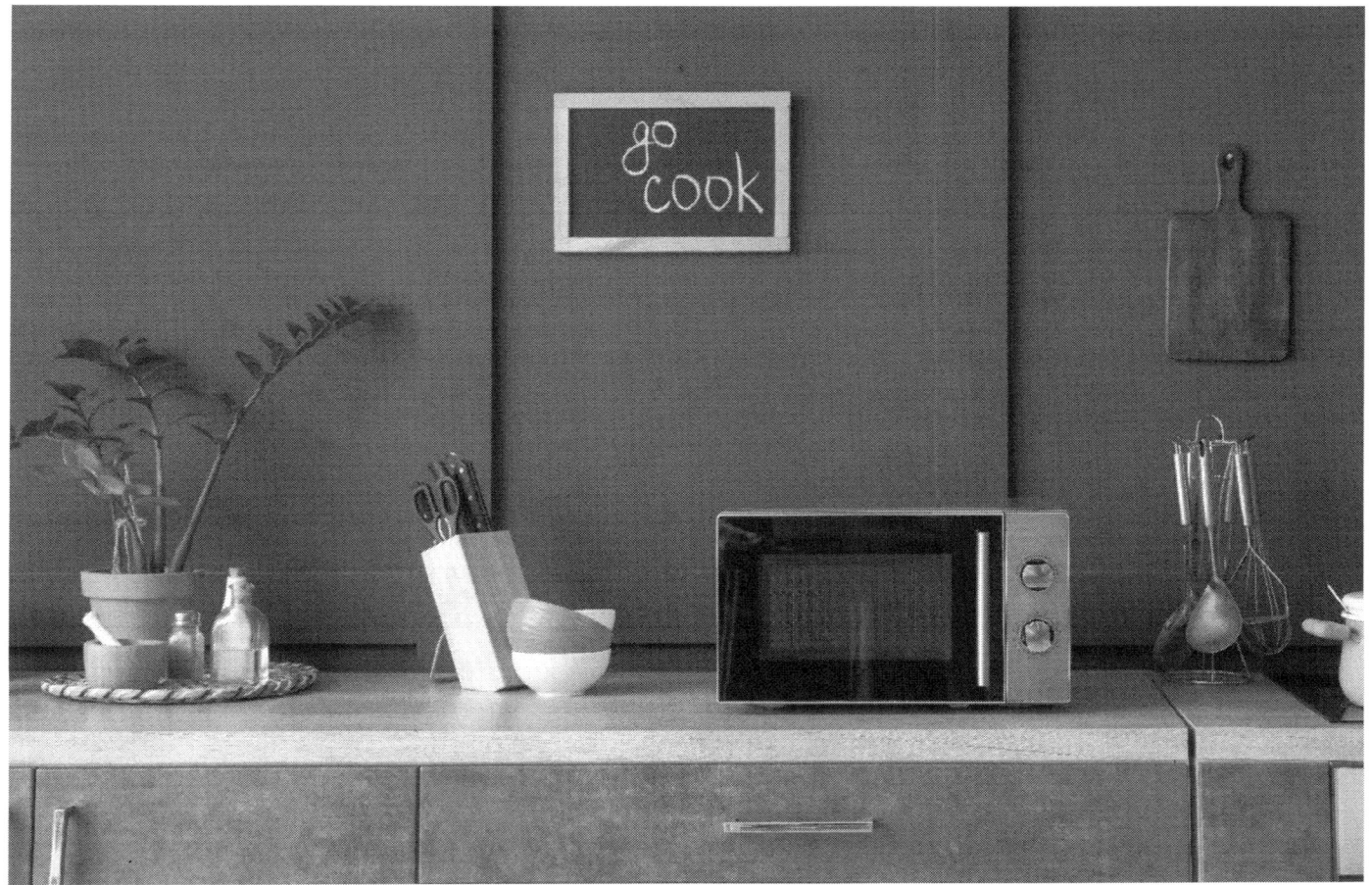

3.1 Basics of Meal Preparation

Understanding the basics of meal preparation is not just a task but the laying of a foundational stone, akin to that of a house, setting the stage for a triumphant nutritional journey that allows you to fuel your body precisely and punctually. This process, meticulous in planning, selection of nutrient-rich ingredients, portion management, and the adoption of efficient cooking and storage practices, morphs meal prep from a mundane task to a rewarding cornerstone of your bodybuilding journey. As we delve deeper, we'll unravel the intricacies of meal prep, offering practical tips, tantalizing recipes, and sustainable strategies, all designed to make this process not just beneficial but enjoyable, aligning seamlessly with your bodybuilding aspirations.

The significance of meal prep cannot be overstated; it's the bedrock of nutritional triumph, ensuring a steady supply of wholesome, balanced meals tailored to your fitness ambitions, circumventing the pitfalls of unhealthy, convenient alternatives. It's a beacon that guides you to optimal energy levels, fortifies muscle recovery, and ensures unwavering adherence to your dietary blueprints. However, the journey begins long before the first pot hits the stove; it starts with meticulous planning. Sketching a detailed meal blueprint for the week, tailored to your nutritional targets, palate preferences, and personal schedule, not only streamlines grocery shopping but also slashes food wastage and banishes the daily culinary conundrum.

The heart of your meal prep lies in the ingredients — a medley of lean proteins, complex carbohydrates, healthy fats, and a rainbow of fruits and vegetables, all teeming with the vital macronutrients and micronutrients that catalyze muscle growth, ignite energy production, and bolster overall health. Yet, the art of portion control is equally crucial, a bulwark against the dietary pitfalls of overindulgence or scant servings. Employ measuring tools to align your meals with your caloric and macronutrient goals, sculpting your body composition with precision.

Your cooking methods should be a marriage of efficiency and preservation, techniques like grilling, baking, steaming, and slow-cooking that lock in nutrients without a time sink, coupled with judicious use of healthful oils. Post-preparation, your culinary creations should be nestled in airtight containers, labeled with preparation dates to guarantee freshness and organized within your refrigerator or freezer for effortless access. Amidst this routine, never let variety fall by the wayside; the spice of life should mingle with your consistent meal prep, inviting an array of recipes, flavors, and cuisines to dance on your tongue, sustaining your nutritional voyage with excitement. Finally, time management is the silent protagonist in your meal prep story; dedicating specific slots for this process, whether a daily ritual or a weekly culinary marathon, weaves meal preparation seamlessly into the tapestry of your life.

3.2 Essential Kitchen Equipment for Efficient Meal Preparation

Equipping your kitchen with essential tools is not merely a matter of convenience but a strategic move akin to a craftsman meticulously organizing his workshop. This foresight streamlines the culinary process, injecting precision and safety into your cooking endeavors, and transforming meal preparation from a chore into a delightful, creative pursuit.

Investing in quality kitchen apparatus isn't an extravagance but a foundational step towards culinary artistry and nutritional triumph, a tangible commitment to forging a path of success and sustainability in your bodybuilding journey.

Imagine the humble chef's knife, not just a utensil but an extension of the chef's hand, sharp and durable, seamlessly transitioning from chopping fruits to dicing proteins, an epitome of versatility that smoothens the meal prep process.

The importance of cutting boards, sturdy sentinels of hygiene, cannot be overstated, safeguarding against cross-contamination by dedicating separate boards for produce and proteins. Precision in the kitchen is not just desirable but essential, achieved through faithful measuring cups and spoons, guardians of accuracy in recipes and portion control, complemented by a kitchen scale, the arbitrator of exactness, especially for proteins. Then, the mixing bowls, a culinary chorus in varying sizes, harmonizing the preparation of salads, marination of proteins, and amalgamation of diverse ingredients. The kitchen's powerhouse, the blender or food processor, stands ready, a maestro of versatility, orchestrating textures and flavors in smoothies, sauces, and soups. Your cookware set, akin to a culinary wardrobe, must boast non-stick, heat-conductive, and durable pieces, offering flexibility across culinary endeavors, while baking sheets and dishes, the workhorses of the kitchen, facilitate everything from roasting vegetables to batch cooking.

Amidst the culinary ballet, the unsung heroes are the airtight containers, steadfast guardians of freshness, ensuring your painstakingly prepared meals remain untainted, whether in the fridge or freezer. For those juggling time, a slow cooker or Instant Pot becomes an invaluable ally, conjuring large meals with minimal fuss, perfect for tender meats and comforting stews. Let's not forget the humble colander and strainer, indispensable for draining, washing, and sifting, or the precision duo of timer and thermometer, ensuring your meals cook accurately and meats reach safe consumption temperatures, respectively. In the realm of culinary convenience, the microwave stands paramount, an essential beacon in meal prepping. More than a reheating conduit, it's a pivotal time-saver, adeptly preserving flavor and nutrients with rapid efficiency, a critical component in maintaining the integrity and deliciousness of meticulously planned meals.

In this symphony of efficiency and creativity, each tool plays a pivotal role, setting the stage for a bodybuilding journey fueled by nutritious, meticulously prepared meals.

Kitchen Conversion

Weight

imperial	metric
1/2 oz	15 g
1 oz	29 g
2 oz	57 g
3 oz	85 g
4 oz	113 g
5 oz	141 g
6 oz	170 g
8 oz	227 g
10 oz	283 g
12 oz	340 g
13 oz	369 g
14 oz	397 g
15 oz	425 g
1 lb	453 g

Measurement

cup	onces	milliliters	tablespoons
8 cup	64 oz	1895 ml	128
6 cup	48 oz	1420 ml	96
5 cup	40 oz	1180 ml	80
4 cup	32 oz	960 ml	64
2 cup	16 oz	480 ml	32
1 cup	8 oz	240 ml	16
3/4 cup	6 oz	177 ml	12
2/3 cup	5 oz	158 ml	11
1/2 cup	4 oz	118 ml	8
3/8 cup	3 oz	90 ml	6
1/3 cup	2.5 oz	79 ml	5.5
1/4 cup	2 oz	59 ml	4
1/8 cup	1 oz	30 ml	3
1/16 cup	1/2 oz	15 ml	1

3.3 Grocery Shopping Essentials

Embarking on a bodybuilding journey demands not just physical rigor but also strategic grocery shopping, with a well-thought-out list as your pivotal ally, ensuring a trove of essential, muscle-fueling ingredients. This begins with a keen focus on proteins, the quintessential building blocks of muscle, necessitating a cart abundant with diverse lean proteins — from staples like chicken breast, turkey, and lean beef to aquatic offerings such as fish and dietary inclusivities like eggs and plant-based stalwarts including lentils and chickpeas. The carbohydrate narrative is selective, championing the complex kind — whole grains like brown rice, quinoa, oats, and steadfast starchy comrades like sweet potatoes and legumes — all curated for the promise of sustained energy. The grocery expedition is incomplete without the strategic alliance of healthy fats, indispensable for hormone orchestration crucial to muscle morphology, making avocados, nuts, seeds, olive oil, and fatty fish non-negotiable cart inclusions.

Amidst this macronutrient symphony, vegetables in their chromatic splendor command attention, their hues a silent testament to their nutrient density, making leafy greens, bell peppers, broccoli, and their colorful kin essential. The fruit section offers nature's candy, with berries, oranges, apples, and bananas doubling as nutrient powerhouses and palate pleasers. Beyond edibles, hydration reigns supreme, with water, herbal teas, and low-calorie beverages being silent heroes in muscle functionality and holistic health.

The shopping saga also embraces prudent snacking, standing as sentinels against untimely hunger. Convenience, especially on frenzied days, finds its place with pre-cut vegetables, canned legumes, and unsweetened frozen produce. This culinary odyssey, though seemingly mundane, is a tactical feat, anchored by a detailed, section-organized shopping list, a shield against impulsive diversions and forgetfulness. It demands label literacy to sieve out hidden sugars, unhealthy fats, and sodium, and champions bulk buying, a nod to economic and environmental mindfulness. This grocery choreography, far from perfunctory, is a deliberate, strategic dance designed for nutritional triumph on the bodybuilding stage.

3.4 Time Management and Scheduling

Time management in bodybuilding is an art of strategic organization, where every second consolidates the foundation for a robust, healthier physique. It begins with the establishment of a routine, a rhythmic cadence that orchestrates the symphony of tasks from grocery shopping to the tranquility of rest, each element synchronized to the grand composition of muscle growth and recovery. Meal preparation stands at the forefront of this regimen, its significance emphasized by dedicated time slots, ensuring that the siren call of convenience and fast food is drowned out by the harmonious melodies of nutritious, home-cooked meals. The kitchen transforms into a stage of efficiency with the introduction of time-saving maestros: pressure cookers, blenders, and food processors, each playing a pivotal role in the culinary ballet of health and fitness.

Moreover, the script of this performance, the meal plan, is meticulously scribed, detailed and precise, precluding the chaos of indecision and fortifying the bastion against nutritional misdemeanors. The grocery shopping saga is no less orchestrated, with a list that mirrors a treasure map, organized not by jewels but by aisles and categories, a path often tread digitally in the realms of online commerce. The culinary act reaches its crescendo in the form of batch cooking, a chorus of meals prepared in harmony, their nutritious refrains resonating throughout the week.

Yet, the composition does not solely confine itself to nutrition; it extends its reach to the sanctuaries of workouts and rest, their allocation as sacred as the meals themselves, all in a delicate balance to nurture muscle and spirit. Amidst this, technology emerges as a silent conductor, its digital baton guiding the rhythm of schedules, motivation, and progress tracking. However, lurking in the shadows, procrastination, a discordant note, threatens the melody, quelled only by the strategic segmentation of tasks and the relentless march of deadlines. In this symphony of bodybuilding, each tick of the clock is a note in a grand opus, each routine a movement towards a magnum opus of physical triumph.

4 Sunrise Fuel for Your Day

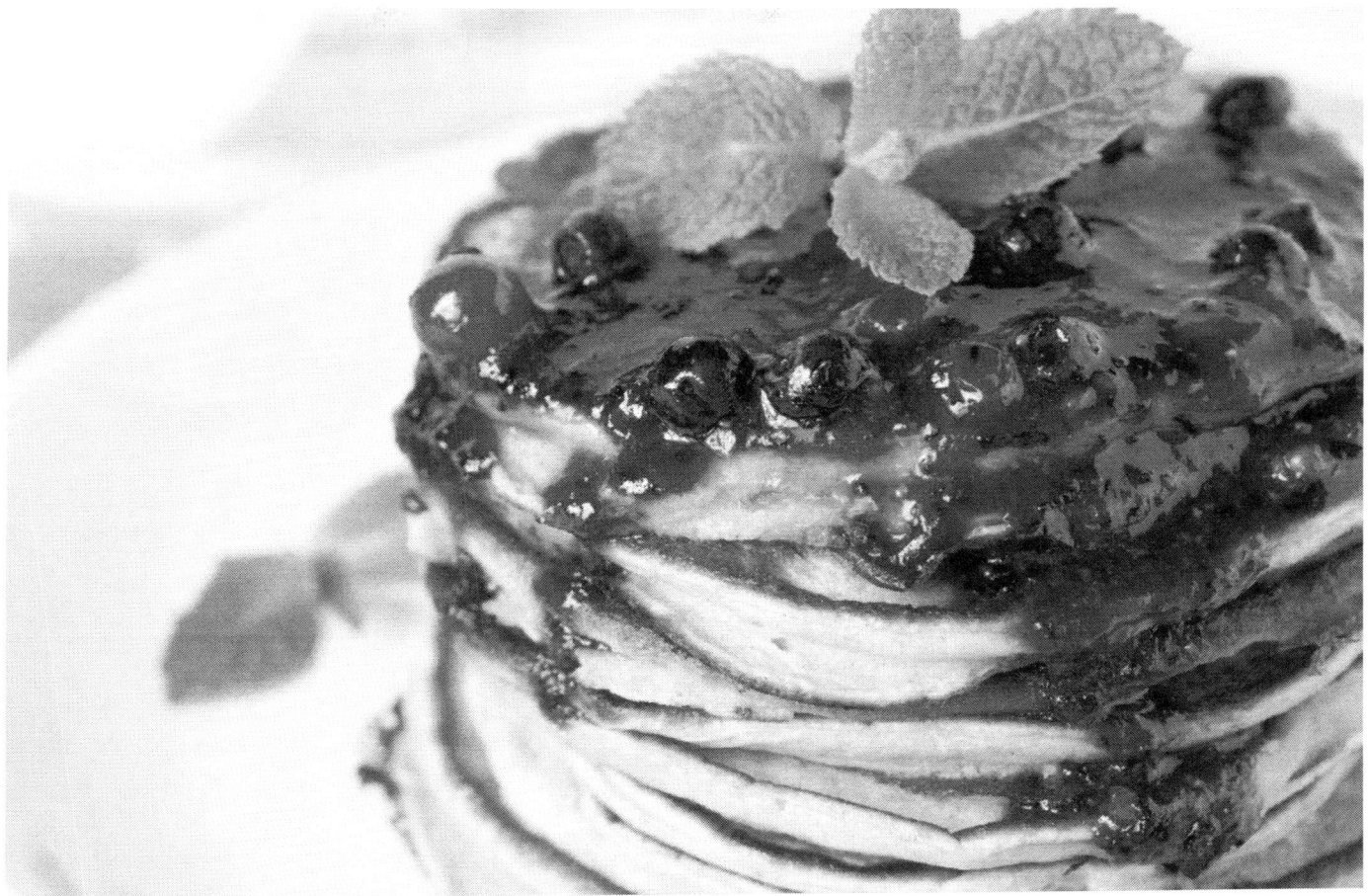

Protein Pancakes with Berry Compote - Page 27

Embarking on a bodybuilding journey necessitates meticulous attention to diet, with breakfast serving as a foundational pillar. Breakfast recipes within a bodybuilding meal prep regimen are meticulously crafted to ignite the metabolism, fuel intense physical training, and initiate daily muscle repair and growth processes.

They're not just meals but strategic tools designed to optimize the body's anabolic environment, proving that in bodybuilding, breakfast is more than a meal—it's the bedrock of success.

Please note: the recipes are designed for one serving, allowing you the freedom to determine the number of meals you prepare in advance. Ensure you examine the food's condition before reheating and discard anything that appears or smells suspicious.

Protein-Packed Oatm

Preparation Time: 5 minutes
Cooking Time: 10 minutes
Servings: 1

Ingredients:
½ cup Rolled Oats
1 cup Water
1 scoop Whey Protein Powder (Vanilla)
½ medium Banana, sliced
1 tbsp Almond Butter
1 tbsp Chia Seeds
A pinch of Salt

Instructions: In a saucepan, bring water to a boil. Add a pinch of salt and oats. Reduce heat to medium and cook for about 5-7 minutes, stirring occasionally. After the oatmeal is cooked, take it from the stove and mix in the protein powder. Top with banana slices, almond butter, and chia seeds.

Nutrient	Amount
Calories	450 kcal
Protein	30g
Total Carbohydrates	45g
- Sugars	15g
- Dietary Fiber	5g
Total Fat	15g
- Saturated Fat	3g

Meal Prepping:

Storage: Store the cooked oatmeal in an airtight container in the refrigerator for up to 5 days.
Keep the toppings (banana, almond butter, chia seeds) separate until you're ready to eat.
Serving: Reheat the oatmeal in a saucepan on the stove or in the microwave, adding a little extra water or milk to achieve your desired consistency.

Egg White & Spinach Scramble

Preparation Time: 5 minutes
Cooking Time: 10 minutes
Servings: 1

Ingredients:
1 cup Egg Whites
1 cup Fresh Spinach, chopped
½ medium Tomato, diced
1 tbsp Feta Cheese, crumbled
Salt and Pepper, to taste
1 tsp Olive Oil

Instructions: Heat olive oil in a non-stick skillet over medium heat. Add the spinach and tomatoes, sautéing until the spinach is wilted. Pour in the egg whites and cook, stirring occasionally, until fully cooked. Season with salt and pepper and top with feta cheese before serving.

Nutrient	Amount
Calories	200 kcal
Protein	30g
Total Carbohydrates	5g
- Sugars	3g
- Dietary Fiber	1g
Total Fat	7g
- Saturated Fat	3g

Meal Prepping:
Storage: Store it in an airtight container in the refrigerator for up to 4 days.
Serving: Reheat the scramble in a skillet over medium heat or in the microwave until warmed through.

Quinoa & Egg Breakfast Bowl

Preparation Time: 10 minutes
Cooking Time: 20 minutes
Servings: 1

Ingredients:
½ cup Cooked Quinoa
2 large Eggs
½ Avocado, sliced
1 cup Mixed Vegetables (e.g. bell peppers, zucchini), diced
Salt and Pepper, to taste
1 tsp Olive Oil

Instructions: In a skillet, heat olive oil over medium heat.
Add the mixed vegetables and sauté until tender.
In another pan, cook the eggs to your preference (scrambled, poached, or fried).
Assemble the bowl with cooked quinoa at the base, topped with vegetables, eggs, and avocado slices.
Season with salt and pepper to taste.

Nutrient	Amount
Calories	450 kcal
Protein	20g
Total Carbohydrates	35g
- Sugars	5g
- Dietary Fiber	8g
Total Fat	25g
- Saturated Fat	5g

Meal Prepping:
Storage: Store the cooked quinoa and sautéed vegetables in an airtight container in the refrigerator for up to 5 days.
Cook the eggs fresh or store them in a separate container in the fridge for up to 2 days.
Serving: Reheat the quinoa and vegetables in the microwave or on the stove.
Serve with the eggs and fresh avocado slices.

Greek Yogurt & Nut Parfait

Preparation Time: 5 minutes
Cooking Time: 0 minutes
Servings: 1

Ingredients:
1 cup Greek Yogurt (non-fat)
1 tbsp Honey
2 tbsp Granola
1 tbsp Almonds, chopped
½ medium Apple, diced

Instructions: In a glass or bowl, layer Greek yogurt with granola, almonds, and diced apple.
Drizzle honey over the top layer.
Serve immediately or refrigerate for later use.

Nutrient	Amount
Calories	350 kcal
Protein	25g
Total Carbohydrates	45g
- Sugars	30g
- Dietary Fiber	5g
Total Fat	10g
- Saturated Fat	2g

Meal Prepping:
<u>Storage:</u> If needed, you can store the yogurt and honey in a container, and the granola, almonds, and apple in separate containers to prevent sogginess. Refrigerate for up to 2 days.
<u>Serving:</u> Assemble the parfait with the stored ingredients and enjoy.

Sweet Potato & Turkey Sausage Hash

Preparation Time: 10 minutes
Cooking Time: 20 minutes
Servings: 1

Ingredients:
1 medium Sweet Potato, diced
3 oz Lean Turkey Sausage, sliced
½ medium Onion, diced
1 cup Kale, chopped
Salt and Pepper, to taste
1 tsp Olive Oil

Instructions: In a skillet, heat olive oil over medium heat.

Add the sweet potato and onion, cooking until the sweet potato is tender.

Add the turkey sausage and cook until browned.

Stir in the kale and cook until wilted.

Season with salt and pepper to taste before serving.

Nutrient	Amount
Calories	400 kcal
Protein	25g
Total Carbohydrates	35g
- Sugars	10g
- Dietary Fiber	5g
Total Fat	15g
- Saturated Fat	4g

Meal Prepping:

Storage: Store it in an airtight container in the refrigerator for up to 4 days.

Serving: Reheat the hash in a skillet over medium heat or in the microwave until hot.

Almond Butter & Banana Smoothie

Preparation Time: 5 minutes
Cooking Time: 0 minutes
Servings: 1

Ingredients:
1 medium Banana
1 tbsp Almond Butter
1 scoop Chocolate Protein Powder
1 cup Almond Milk (unsweetened)
Ice cubes (optional)

Instructions: Combine all ingredients in a blender.
Blend on high until smooth.
Pour into a glass and enjoy immediately.

Nutrient	Amount
Calories	350 kcal
Protein	25g
Total Carbohydrates	35g
- Sugars	20g
- Dietary Fiber	5g
Total Fat	12g
- Saturated Fat	2g

Meal Prepping:
Storage: Store the ingredients portioned in an airtight container in the freezer for up to a month.
Serving: blend the ingredients with almond milk and enjoy immediately.

Veggie & Egg White Muffins

Preparation Time: 10 minutes
Cooking Time: 20 minutes
Servings: 1

Ingredients:
1 cup Mixed Vegetables (e.g. bell peppers, spinach), chopped
1 cup Egg Whites
Salt and Pepper, to taste
1 tbsp Feta Cheese, crumbled

Instructions: Preheat oven to 350°F (180°C).
In a bowl, mix vegetables, egg whites, salt, and pepper.
Pour the mixture into muffin tins and top with feta cheese.
Bake for 20 minutes or until the eggs are set.

Nutrient	Amount
Calories	200 kcal
Protein	25g
Total Carbohydrates	15g
- Sugars	5g
- Dietary Fiber	3g
Total Fat	5g
- Saturated Fat	1g

Meal Prepping:
Storage: Store the muffins in an airtight container in the refrigerator for up to 4 days or freeze for up to 1 month.
Serving: Reheat the muffins in the microwave or covered in the oven until warm.

Protein Pancakes with Berry Compote

Preparation Time: 10 minutes
Cooking Time: 15 minutes
Servings: 1

Ingredients:
½ cup Oat Flour
1 scoop Vanilla Protein Powder
1 large Egg
½ cup Almond Milk
½ tsp Baking Powder
1 cup Mixed Berries
1 tbsp Maple Syrup
1 tsp Coconut Oil

Instructions: In a bowl, mix oat flour, protein powder, egg, almond milk, and baking powder until smooth.

Heat coconut oil in a non-stick skillet over medium heat.

Pour batter to form pancakes, cooking until bubbles form on the surface, then flip and cook the other side.

In another pan, heat mixed berries and maple syrup over medium heat until berries are soft and syrupy.

Serve pancakes topped with berry compote.

Nutrient	Amount
Calories	450 kcal
Protein	30g
Total Carbohydrates	55g
- Sugars	20g
- Dietary Fiber	8g
Total Fat	12g
- Saturated Fat	5g

Meal Prepping:
Storage: Store the pancakes in an airtight container in the refrigerator for up to 5 days or freeze for up to 2 months.
Store the berry compote in a separate airtight container in the refrigerator for up to 5 days.
Serving: Reheat the pancakes in a toaster, oven, or microwave until warmed through.
Warm the berry compote on the stove or in the microwave until heated to your liking.

Chia Seed & Berry Pudding

Preparation Time: 5 minutes

Cooking Time: 0 minutes

Servings: 1

Ingredients:
2 tbsp Chia Seeds
1 cup Almond Milk (unsweetened)
½ cup Mixed Berries
1 tbsp Honey

Instructions: In a bowl, mix chia seeds and almond milk. Refrigerate for at least 2 hours or overnight until it forms a pudding-like consistency. Top with mixed berries and drizzle with honey before serving.

Nutrient	Amount
Calories	250 kcal
Protein	7g
Total Carbohydrates	35g
- Sugars	20g
- Dietary Fiber	10g
Total Fat	10g
- Saturated Fat	1g

Meal Prepping:

Storage: Store the pancakes in an airtight container in the refrigerator for up to 5 days.

Serving: Top with fresh berries and a drizzle of honey before serving.

Protein French Toast

Preparation Time: 10 minutes
Cooking Time: 10 minutes
Servings: 1

Ingredients:
- 2 slices Whole Grain Bread
- 1 large Egg
- ½ cup Almond Milk (unsweetened)
- 1 scoop Vanilla Protein Powder
- 1 tsp Cinnamon
- 1 tbsp Maple Syrup
- 1 tsp Coconut Oil

Instructions: In a bowl, whisk together egg, almond milk, protein powder, and cinnamon.

Dip each slice of bread into the mixture, ensuring both sides are coated.

Heat coconut oil in a skillet over medium heat.

Cook each slice until golden brown on both sides.

Serve with maple syrup.

Nutrient	Amount
Calories	450 kcal
Protein	30g
Total Carbohydrates	45g
- Sugars	15g
- Dietary Fiber	5g
Total Fat	15g
- Saturated Fat	5g

Meal Prepping:

Storage: Store in an airtight container in the refrigerator for up to 2 days or freeze for up to 1 month.

Serving: Reheat in a toaster oven or in a skillet over medium heat.

Serve with maple syrup.

Quinoa & Berry Breakfast Bowl

Preparation Time: 10 minutes

Cooking Time: 20 minutes

Servings: 1

Ingredients:
- ½ cup Cooked Quinoa
- 1 cup Mixed Berries
- 1 tbsp Almonds, chopped
- 1 tbsp Honey
- 1 scoop Vanilla Protein Powder

Instructions: In a bowl, mix cooked quinoa with protein powder. Top with mixed berries and chopped almonds. Drizzle with honey before serving.

Nutrient	Amount
Calories	400 kcal
Protein	30g
Total Carbohydrates	55g
- Sugars	20g
- Dietary Fiber	7g
Total Fat	10g
- Saturated Fat	1g

Meal Prepping:

<u>Storage:</u> Store in an airtight container in the refrigerator for up to 5 days. Keep berries and almonds separate to maintain freshness and texture.

<u>Serving:</u> Warm the quinoa if desired, then top with fresh berries, almonds, and a drizzle of honey.

Mango & Greek Yogurt Smoothie

Preparation Time: 5 minutes
Cooking Time: 0 minutes
Servings: 1

Ingredients:
1 cup Mango, diced
1 cup Greek Yogurt (non-fat)
1 scoop Vanilla Protein Powder
Ice cubes (optional)

Instructions: Combine all ingredients in a blender.
Blend on high until smooth.
Pour into a glass and enjoy immediately.

Nutrient	Amount
Calories	350 kcal
Protein	35g
Total Carbohydrates	45g
- Sugars	40g
- Dietary Fiber	3g
Total Fat	5g
- Saturated Fat	1g

Meal Prepping:

Storage: Store the pancakes in an airtight container in the refrigerator for up to 5 days or freeze for up to 1 month.

Serving: Blend the frozen ingredients with Greek yogurt until smooth and enjoy immediately.

Veggie & Egg Breakfast Burrito

Preparation Time: 10 minutes
Cooking Time: 15 minutes
Servings: 1

Ingredients:
1 Whole Wheat Tortilla
2 large Eggs, scrambled
1 cup Mixed Vegetables (e.g. bell peppers, onions), diced
½ medium Avocado, sliced
1 tbsp Salsa
Salt and Pepper, to taste
1 tsp Olive Oil

Instructions: In a skillet, heat olive oil over medium heat.
Add the mixed vegetables and sauté until tender.
Add the scrambled eggs and cook until fully cooked.
Lay the tortilla flat and arrange the cooked vegetables and eggs in the center.
Top with avocado slices and salsa.
Roll up the tortilla tightly and cut in half diagonally before serving.

Nutrient	Amount
Calories	450 kcal
Protein	20g
Total Carbohydrates	35g
- Sugars	5g
- Dietary Fiber	7g
Total Fat	25g
- Saturated Fat	5g

Meal Prepping:
Storage: Wrap tightly in aluminum foil. Store in the refrigerator for up to 1 day or freeze for up to 1 month.
Serving: If refrigerated, reheat in the microwave or in a skillet over medium heat. If frozen, thaw in the refrigerator overnight before reheating.

Apple & Cinnamon Oatmeal

Preparation Time: 5 minutes

Cooking Time: 10 minutes

Servings: 1

Ingredients:
- ½ cup Rolled Oats
- 1 cup Water
- ½ medium Apple, diced
- 1 tbsp Almonds, chopped
- 1 tsp Cinnamon
- 1 tbsp Maple Syrup
- A pinch of Salt

Instructions: In a saucepan, bring water to a boil. Add a pinch of salt and oats. Reduce heat to medium and cook for about 5-7 minutes, stirring occasionally. Once the oats are cooked, remove from heat and stir in the cinnamon and maple syrup. Top with diced apple and chopped almonds before serving.

Nutrient	Amount
Calories	350 kcal
Protein	10g
Total Carbohydrates	55g
- Sugars	25g
- Dietary Fiber	7g
Total Fat	10g
- Saturated Fat	1g

Meal Prepping:

Storage: Store in an airtight container in the refrigerator for up to 5 days.

Keep the apple and almonds separate until ready to serve.

Serving: Reheat the oatmeal on the stove or in the microwave, adding extra water or milk if needed.

Top with fresh apple and almonds, then serve.

Protein-Packed Muesli

Preparation Time: 5 minutes

Cooking Time: 0 minutes

Servings: 1

Ingredients:
½ cup Muesli
1 scoop Vanilla Protein Powder
1 cup Almond Milk (unsweetened)
½ medium Banana, sliced
1 tbsp Almonds, chopped

Instructions: In a bowl, mix muesli with protein powder. Pour almond milk over the mixture and stir well. Top with banana slices and chopped almonds before serving.

Nutrient	Amount
Calories	400 kcal
Protein	30g
Total Carbohydrates	45g
- Sugars	20g
- Dietary Fiber	5g
Total Fat	12g
- Saturated Fat	2g

Meal Prepping:

Storage: Mix the muesli with protein powder and store in an airtight container in a cool, dry place for up to a week.
Store the almond milk in the refrigerator and add when ready to serve.

Serving: Pour almond milk over the muesli mixture, then top with fresh banana slices and almonds.

5 Satisfying Lunchtime Delights to Recharge

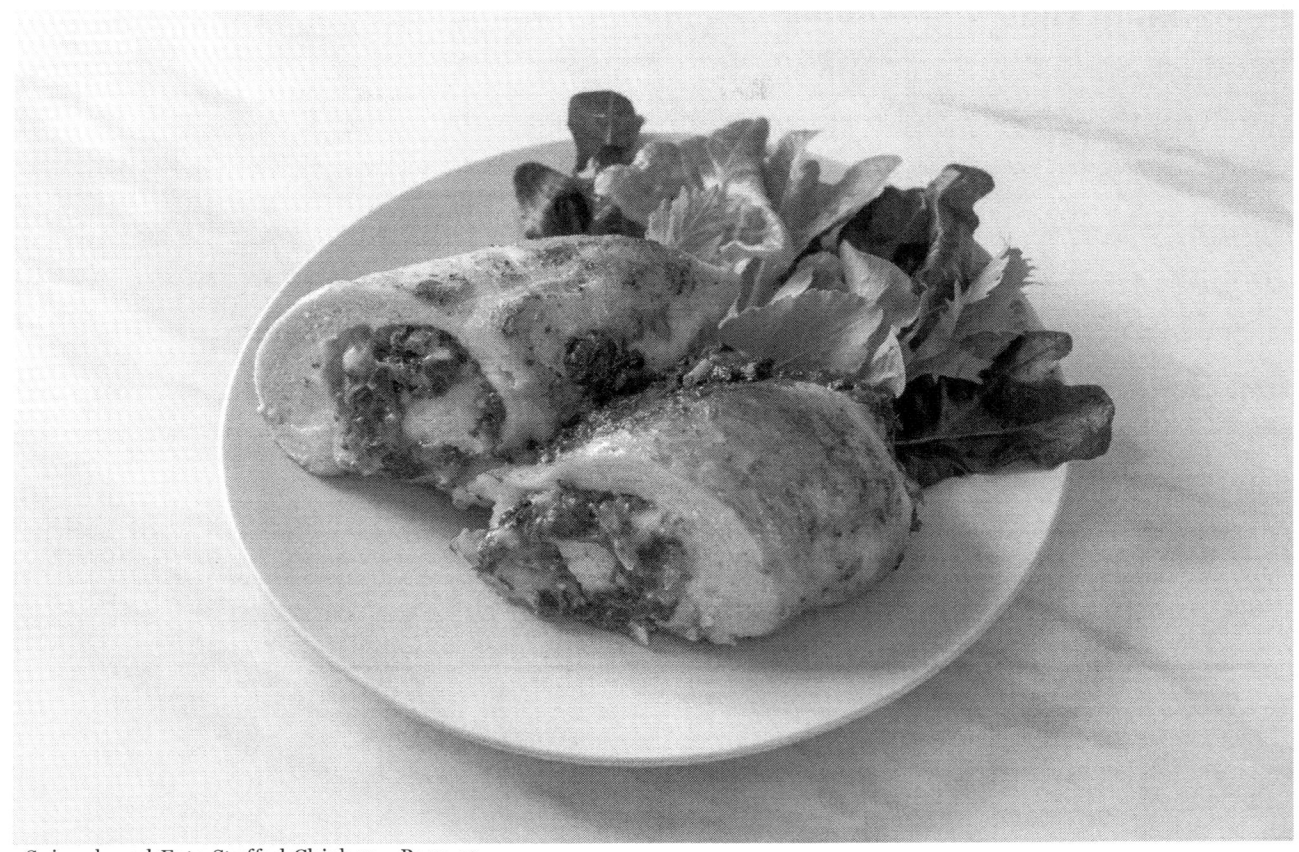

Spinach and Feta Stuffed Chicken - Page 43

In the realm of bodybuilding, lunch is more than a midday meal; it's a critical opportunity to continue fueling the body's muscle-building processes initiated during breakfast. Lunch recipes in bodybuilding meal prep focus on a balanced integration of protein, complex carbohydrates, and essential fats, all crucial for sustained energy, optimal muscle repair, and growth throughout the day.

They underscore the principle that in bodybuilding, every meal is an opportunity to nourish the body and edge closer to one's physical goals.

Please note: the recipes are designed for one serving, allowing you the freedom to determine the number of meals you prepare in advance. Ensure you examine the food's condition before reheating and discard anything that appears or smells suspicious.

Grilled Chicken & Quinoa Salad

Preparation Time: 10 minutes
Cooking Time: 15 minutes
Servings: 1

Ingredients:
6 oz Chicken Breast
½ cup Cooked Quinoa
1 cup Mixed Greens
½ medium Avocado, sliced
1 tbsp Olive Oil
Salt and Pepper, to taste
1 tbsp Balsamic Vinaigrette

Instructions: Season chicken breast with salt and pepper. Grill over medium heat until fully cooked. In a bowl, mix quinoa, mixed greens, and avocado. Drizzle with olive oil and balsamic vinaigrette before serving.

Nutrient	Amount
Calories	500 kcal
Protein	40g
Total Carbohydrates	35g
- Sugars	5g
- Dietary Fiber	8g
Total Fat	25g
- Saturated Fat	4g

Meal Prepping:
Storage: Store the salad in an airtight container in the refrigerator for up to 3-4 days.
Store the dressing separately.
Serving: Drizzle with dressing just before serving.

Turkey & Veggie Skillet

Preparation Time: 10 minutes
Cooking Time: 20 minutes
Servings: 1

Ingredients:
6 oz Ground Turkey
1 cup Mixed Vegetables (e.g. bell peppers, zucchini), diced
1 tbsp Olive Oil
Salt and Pepper, to taste
1 tsp Paprika

Instructions: In a skillet, heat olive oil over medium heat. Add ground turkey and cook until browned. Add vegetables, salt, pepper, and paprika. Sauté until vegetables are tender.

Nutrient	Amount
Calories	400 kcal
Protein	35g
Total Carbohydrates	25g
- Sugars	6g
- Dietary Fiber	6g
Total Fat	20g
- Saturated Fat	4g

Meal Prepping:
Storage: Store in an airtight container in the refrigerator for up to 3-4 days.
Serving: Reheat on the stove over medium heat, stirring occasionally, or in the microwave until warmed through.

Spicy Tuna Salad

Preparation Time: 10 minutes
Cooking Time: 0 minutes
Servings: 1

Ingredients:
1 can (5 oz) Tuna in Water, drained
1 cup Mixed Greens
½ medium Avocado, diced
1 tbsp Olive Oil
1 tbsp Lemon Juice
Salt and Pepper, to taste
½ tsp Crushed Red Pepper Flakes

Instructions: In a bowl, mix tuna, mixed greens, and avocado. Drizzle with olive oil and lemon juice. Season with salt, pepper, and red pepper flakes before serving.

Nutrient	Amount
Calories	350 kcal
Protein	30g
Total Carbohydrates	15g
- Sugars	3g
- Dietary Fiber	7g
Total Fat	20g
- Saturated Fat	3g

Meal Prepping:

Storage: Store the salad ingredients separately in different compartments or containers in the refrigerator for up to 2-3 days.

Do not mix until you're ready to eat.

Serving: Combine ingredients, drizzle with the dressing, and serve.

Classic Grilled Chicken Salad

Preparation Time: 10 minutes
Cooking Time: 15 minutes
Servings: 1

Ingredients:
6 oz Chicken breast
2 cups Mixed salad greens
10 pieces Cherry tomatoes
½ Cucumber, sliced
1 oz Feta cheese:
1 tbsp Olive oil
1 tbsp Lemon juice
Salt and pepper, to taste

Instructions: Season the chicken breast with salt and pepper. Grill until fully cooked.
In a bowl, mix salad greens, cherry tomatoes, and cucumber.
Slice the grilled chicken and place it on top of the salad.
Drizzle with olive oil and lemon juice. Top with feta cheese.

Nutrient	Amount
Calories	400 kcal
Protein	40g
Total Carbohydrates	10g
- Sugars	4g
- Dietary Fiber	3g
Total Fat	20g
- Saturated Fat	4g

Meal Prepping:
Storage: Store the chicken sliced and other salad ingredients separately in the refrigerator for up to 3-4 days.
Till you're ready to dine, keep the dressing separate.
Serving: Assemble the salad, top with sliced chicken, and drizzle with dressing.

Sweet Potato & Black Bean Bowl

Preparation Time: 10 minutes
Cooking Time: 20 minutes
Servings: 1

Ingredients:
1 medium Sweet Potato, diced
½ cup Black Beans, cooked
1 cup Quinoa, cooked
1 tbsp Olive Oil
Salt and Pepper, to taste
1 tbsp Salsa

Instructions: In a skillet, heat olive oil over medium heat. Add sweet potato and cook until tender. In a bowl, mix sweet potato, black beans, and quinoa. Season with salt and pepper, and top with salsa before serving.

Nutrient	Amount
Calories	450 kcal
Protein	20g
Total Carbohydrates	65g
- Sugars	8g
- Dietary Fiber	12g
Total Fat	15g
- Saturated Fat	2g

Meal Prepping:

Storage: Store in an airtight container in the refrigerator for up to 3-4 days.

Serving: Reheat in the microwave or on the stove until warmed through.

Spiced Lentil and Chicken Soup

Preparation Time: 10 minutes
Cooking Time: 30 minutes
Servings: 1

Ingredients:
4 oz Chicken breasts, diced
½ cup Lentils
2 cups Chicken broth
½ tsp Cumin
½ tsp Turmeric
½ tsp Paprika
1 tbsp Olive oil
Salt and pepper, to taste

Instructions: In a pot, heat olive oil and add diced chicken. Cook until browned.
Add lentils, spices, and chicken broth. Bring to a boil.
Reduce heat and let simmer for 20-25 minutes or until lentils are tender.
Season with salt and pepper.

Nutrient	Amount
Calories	400 kcal
Protein	40g
Total Carbohydrates	40g
- Sugars	3g
- Dietary Fiber	10g
Total Fat	10g
- Saturated Fat	2g

Meal Prepping:
Storage: Store in an airtight container in the refrigerator for up to 4-5 days or freeze for up to 6 months.
Serving: Reheat on the stove over medium heat, stirring occasionally, or in the microwave until hot.

Veggie & Quinoa Stir-Fry

Preparation Time: 10 minutes

Cooking Time: 20 minutes

Servings: 1

Ingredients:
- 1 cup Mixed Vegetables (e.g. bell peppers, broccoli), diced
- ½ cup Cooked Quinoa
- 1 tbsp Olive Oil
- 1 tbsp Soy Sauce (low sodium)
- 1 tsp Ginger, grated
- 1 Garlic Clove, minced

Instructions: In a skillet, heat olive oil over medium heat. Add mixed vegetables and sauté until tender. Add cooked quinoa, soy sauce, ginger, and garlic. Stir-fry for a few minutes before serving.

Nutrient	Amount
Calories	350 kcal
Protein	10g
Total Carbohydrates	45g
- Sugars	5g
- Dietary Fiber	8g
Total Fat	15g
- Saturated Fat	2g

Meal Prepping:

<u>Storage:</u> Store in an airtight container in the refrigerator for up to 3-4 days.

<u>Serving:</u> Reheat on the stove over medium heat, stirring occasionally, or in the microwave until warmed through.

Spinach and Feta Stuffed Chicken

Preparation Time: 15 minutes
Cooking Time: 25 minutes
Servings: 1

Ingredients:
6 oz Chicken breast
1 cup Fresh spinach
1 oz Feta cheese
1 tbsp Olive oil
1 clove Garlic, minced
Salt and pepper, to taste

Instructions: Preheat oven to 375°F (190°C).

In a pan, heat ½ tbsp olive oil and sauté garlic and spinach until wilted.

Make a slit in the chicken breast and stuff with spinach and feta.

Season with salt and pepper. Drizzle with remaining olive oil.

Bake for 25 minutes or until chicken is fully cooked.

Nutrient	Amount
Calories	400 kcal
Protein	40g
Total Carbohydrates	5g
- Sugars	1g
- Dietary Fiber	1g
Total Fat	24g
- Saturated Fat	6g

Meal Prepping:

Storage: Store in an airtight container in the refrigerator for up to 3-4 days.

Serving: Reheat in a preheated oven at 350°F (175°C) for about 10-15 minutes or until heated through.

Spicy Chicken & Rice Bowl

Preparation Time: 10 minutes
Cooking Time: 20 minutes
Servings: 1

Ingredients:
6 oz Chicken Breast, diced
½ cup Brown Rice, cooked
1 cup Mixed Vegetables (e.g. bell peppers, onions), diced
1 tbsp Olive Oil
Salt and Pepper, to taste
½ tsp Crushed Red Pepper Flakes

Instructions: In a skillet, heat olive oil over medium heat.
Add chicken and cook until fully cooked.
Add mixed vegetables and sauté until tender.
Mix in cooked rice, salt, pepper, and red pepper flakes before serving.

Nutrient	Amount
Calories	450 kcal
Protein	40g
Total Carbohydrates	45g
- Sugars	3g
- Dietary Fiber	4g
Total Fat	15g
- Saturated Fat	3g

Meal Prepping:
Storage: Store in an airtight container in the refrigerator for up to 3-4 days.
Serving: Reheat in the microwave or on the stove until warmed through, stirring occasionally.

Beef & Sweet Potato Hash

Preparation Time: 10 minutes
Cooking Time: 20 minutes
Servings: 1

Ingredients:
6 oz Lean Ground Beef
1 medium Sweet Potato, diced
1 tbsp Olive Oil
Salt and Pepper, to taste
1 tsp Paprika

Instructions: In a skillet, heat olive oil over medium heat.
Add ground beef and cook until browned.
Add sweet potato and cook until tender.
Season with salt, pepper, and paprika before serving.

Nutrient	Amount
Calories	450 kcal
Protein	35g
Total Carbohydrates	35g
- Sugars	7g
- Dietary Fiber	5g
Total Fat	20g
- Saturated Fat	6g

Meal Prepping:
Storage: Store in an airtight container in the refrigerator for up to 3-4 days.
Serving: Reheat on the stove over medium heat, stirring occasionally, or in the microwave until warmed through.

Turkey & Veggie Lettuce Wraps

Preparation Time: 10 minutes

Cooking Time: 15 minutes

Servings: 1

Ingredients:

6 oz Ground Turkey

1 cup Mixed Vegetables (e.g. bell peppers, carrots), diced

4 Lettuce Leaves

1 tbsp Olive Oil

Salt and Pepper, to taste

1 tbsp Soy Sauce (low sodium)

Instructions: In a skillet, heat olive oil over medium heat.

Add ground turkey and cook until browned.

Add mixed vegetables and sauté until tender.

Spoon the mixture into lettuce leaves and drizzle with soy sauce before serving.

Nutrient	Amount
Calories	400 kcal
Protein	35g
Total Carbohydrates	25g
- Sugars	5g
- Dietary Fiber	6g
Total Fat	20g
- Saturated Fat	4g

Meal Prepping:

Storage: Store in an airtight container in the refrigerator for up to 3-4 days.

Keep lettuce leaves fresh in a ziplock bag with a paper towel.

Serving: Reheat the turkey and veggie mixture, spoon into lettuce leaves, drizzle with soy sauce, and serve.

Salmon & Veggie Skewers

Preparation Time: 10 minutes
Cooking Time: 15 minutes
Servings: 1

Ingredients:
6 oz Salmon Fillet, cut into chunks
1 cup Mixed Vegetables (e.g. bell peppers, zucchini), cut into chunks
1 tbsp Olive Oil
Salt and Pepper, to taste
1 Lemon Slice

Instructions: Preheat grill to medium heat.
Thread salmon and vegetable chunks onto skewers.
Drizzle with olive oil and season with salt and pepper.
Grill until salmon is cooked through, turning occasionally.
Serve with a lemon slice.

Nutrient	Amount
Calories	350 kcal
Protein	35g
Total Carbohydrates	15g
- Sugars	3g
- Dietary Fiber	2g
Total Fat	20g
- Saturated Fat	3g

Meal Prepping:

Storage: Store in an airtight container in the refrigerator for up to 2-3 days.

Serving: Reheat in the oven on a baking sheet at 350°F (175°C) for about 10 minutes or until heated through.

Chicken & Veggie Pasta

Preparation Time: 10 minutes
Cooking Time: 20 minutes
Servings: 1

Ingredients:
6 oz Chicken Breast, sliced
1 cup Whole Wheat Pasta, cooked
1 cup Mixed Vegetables (e.g. cherry tomatoes, spinach)
1 tbsp Olive Oil
Salt and Pepper, to taste
1 tbsp Parmesan Cheese, grated

Instructions: In a skillet, cook chicken slices until fully cooked.
Add mixed vegetables and sauté until tender.
Mix in cooked pasta, olive oil, salt, and pepper.
Top with parmesan cheese before serving.

Nutrient	Amount
Calories	450 kcal
Protein	40g
Total Carbohydrates	45g
- Sugars	4g
- Dietary Fiber	6g
Total Fat	15g
- Saturated Fat	3g

Meal Prepping:

Storage: Store in an airtight container in the refrigerator for up to 3-4 days.

Serving: Reheat in the microwave or on the stove, adding a little water or broth to prevent dryness, until warmed through.

Beef & Veggie Stir-Fry

Preparation Time: 10 minutes
Cooking Time: 15 minutes
Servings: 1

Ingredients:
6 oz Lean Beef Strips
1 cup Mixed Vegetables (e.g. bell peppers, snap peas), sliced
1 tbsp Olive Oil
1 tbsp Soy Sauce (low sodium)
1 tsp Ginger, grated
1 Garlic Clove, minced

Instructions: In a skillet, heat olive oil over medium heat. Add beef strips and cook until browned. Add mixed vegetables, soy sauce, ginger, and garlic. Stir-fry until vegetables are tender.

Nutrient	Amount
Calories	400 kcal
Protein	35g
Total Carbohydrates	25g
- Sugars	5g
- Dietary Fiber	5g
Total Fat	20g
- Saturated Fat	5g

Meal Prepping:
Storage: Store the stir-fry in an airtight container in the refrigerator for up to 3-4 days.
Serving: Reheat on the stove over medium heat, stirring occasionally, or in the microwave until warmed through.

Chickpea and Quinoa Salad

Preparation Time: 10 minutes

Cooking Time: 20 minutes

Servings: 1

Ingredients:
- ½ cup Quinoa
- ½ cup Chickpeas, cooked
- ½ Cucumber, diced
- ½ Red bell pepper, diced
- 1 tbsp Olive oil
- 1 tbsp Lemon juice
- 1 tbsp Fresh parsley, chopped
- Salt and pepper, to taste

Instructions: Cook quinoa as per package instructions.

In a bowl, mix quinoa, chickpeas, cucumber, and red bell pepper.

Drizzle with olive oil and lemon juice. Mix well and garnish with fresh parsley.

Nutrient	Amount
Calories	400 kcal
Protein	15g
Total Carbohydrates	55g
- Sugars	8g
- Dietary Fiber	10g
Total Fat	15g
- Saturated Fat	2g

Meal Prepping:

Storage: Store the salad in an airtight container in the refrigerator for up to 3-4 days.

For best results, add the dressing and parsley just before serving.

Serving: Stir the salad well and serve cold or at room temperature.

Shrimp & Veggie Salad

Preparation Time: 10 minutes
Cooking Time: 10 minutes
Servings: 1

Ingredients:
6 oz Shrimp, peeled and deveined
1 cup Mixed Greens
1 cup Mixed Vegetables (e.g. cherry tomatoes, cucumbers), diced
1 tbsp Olive Oil
1 tbsp Lemon Juice
Salt and Pepper, to taste

Instructions: In a skillet, cook shrimp until pink.
In a bowl, mix shrimp, mixed greens, and mixed vegetables.
Drizzle with olive oil and lemon juice.
Season with salt and pepper before serving.

Nutrient	Amount
Calories	350 kcal
Protein	35g
Total Carbohydrates	25g
- Sugars	4g
- Dietary Fiber	5g
Total Fat	15g
- Saturated Fat	2g

Meal Prepping:
Storage: Store the shrimp separately from the greens and veggies in the refrigerator for up to 2 days.
Store the dressing separately.
Serving: Combine shrimp, greens, and veggies, drizzle with dressing, and serve.

Classic Grilled Chicken Quinoa Tabbouleh

Preparation Time: 15 minutes
Cooking Time: 15 minutes
Servings: 1

Ingredients:
4 oz chicken breast
½ cup cooked quinoa
¼ cup cherry tomatoes, halved
¼ cup cucumber, diced
¼ cup bell peppers, diced
¼ cup chickpeas, cooked
1 tbsp olive oil
Salt and pepper, to taste
Fresh herbs (parsley, mint), chopped
Lemon juice, to taste

Instructions: Preheat the grill to medium-high heat. Season the chicken with salt, pepper, and a drizzle of olive oil. Grill until fully cooked, approximately 7 minutes per side. Let it rest for a few minutes, then slice.

In a bowl, combine the cooked quinoa, cherry tomatoes, cucumber, bell peppers, and chickpeas.

Add the chopped herbs, olive oil, lemon juice, salt, and pepper to the quinoa mixture. Toss to combine.

Serve the tabbouleh topped with grilled chicken slices.

Nutrient	Amount
Calories	400 kcal
Protein	35g
Total Carbohydrates	30g
- Sugars	5g
- Dietary Fiber	6g
Total Fat	15g
- Saturated Fat	2g

Meal Prepping:

<u>Storage:</u> Store the grilled chicken and quinoa mixture separately in airtight containers in the refrigerator for up to 3-4 days.

<u>Serving:</u> Reheat the chicken in a microwave or on a stovetop until it's warmed through. Be careful not to overcook it.

The quinoa tabbouleh can be eaten cold or slightly warmed in the microwave.

Serve the tabbouleh topped with the grilled chicken slices.

Chicken & Veggie Kabobs

Preparation Time: 10 minutes
Cooking Time: 15 minutes
Servings: 1

Ingredients:
6 oz Chicken Breast, cut into chunks
1 cup Mixed Vegetables (e.g. bell peppers, zucchini), cut into chunks
1 tbsp Olive Oil
Salt and Pepper, to taste
1 Lemon Slice

Instructions: Preheat grill to medium heat. Thread chicken and vegetable chunks onto skewers. Drizzle with olive oil and season with salt and pepper. Grill until chicken is cooked through, turning occasionally. Serve with a lemon slice.

Nutrient	Amount
Calories	350 kcal
Protein	40g
Total Carbohydrates	15g
- Sugars	3g
- Dietary Fiber	4g
Total Fat	15g
- Saturated Fat	3g

Meal Prepping:
Storage: Store in an airtight container in the refrigerator for up to 3-4 days.
Serving: Reheat on a baking sheet in the oven at 350°F (175°C) for about 10 minutes or until heated through.

Beef & Veggie Bowl

Preparation Time: 10 minutes
Cooking Time: 15 minutes
Servings: 1

Ingredients:
6 oz Lean Beef Strips
1 cup Mixed Vegetables (e.g. bell peppers, snap peas), sliced
½ cup Quinoa, cooked
1 tbsp Olive Oil
Salt and Pepper, to taste
1 tbsp Soy Sauce (low sodium)

Instructions: In a skillet, heat olive oil over medium heat.
Add beef strips and cook until browned.
Add mixed vegetables and sauté until tender.
Mix in cooked quinoa, salt, pepper, and soy sauce before serving.

Nutrient	Amount
Calories	450 kcal
Protein	35g
Total Carbohydrates	45g
- Sugars	5g
- Dietary Fiber	6g
Total Fat	20g
- Saturated Fat	6g

Meal Prepping:

Storage: Store in an airtight container in the refrigerator for up to 3-4 days.

Serving: Reheat in the microwave or in a skillet over medium heat until warmed through.

Pesto Grilled Shrimp Quinoa Bowl

Preparation Time: 15 minutes
Cooking Time: 20 minutes
Servings: 1

Ingredients:
6 oz Large shrimp, peeled and deveined
½ cup cooked Quinoa
2 tbsp Pesto sauce
6-8 Cherry tomatoes, halved
1 tbsp Olive oil
1 Lemon wedge

Instructions: Marinate the shrimp in pesto sauce for 10 minutes.

In a pan, heat olive oil and grill the shrimp until pink and fully cooked.

Serve the shrimp over cooked quinoa, add cherry tomatoes, and squeeze a lemon wedge over the top.

Nutrient	Amount
Calories	400 kcal
Protein	35g
Total Carbohydrates	40g
- Sugars	3g
- Dietary Fiber	5g
Total Fat	15g
- Saturated Fat	3g

Meal Prepping:

Storage: Store the shrimp separately from the cooked quinoa and tomatoes in an airtight container in the refrigerator for up to 2 days.

Serving: Serve the shrimp over quinoa, add tomatoes, and squeeze a lemon wedge over the top. Best enjoyed cold or at room temperature.

Spicy Tuna & Veggie Wrap

Preparation Time: 10 minutes
Cooking Time: 0 minutes
Servings: 1

Ingredients:
1 can (5 oz) Tuna in Water, drained
1 Whole Wheat Tortilla
1 cup Mixed Vegetables (e.g. bell peppers, spinach), sliced
1 tbsp Greek Yogurt
Salt and Pepper, to taste
½ tsp Crushed Red Pepper Flakes

Instructions: In a bowl, mix tuna, Greek yogurt, salt, pepper, and red pepper flakes. Lay the tortilla flat and arrange tuna mixture and mixed vegetables in the center. Roll up the tortilla tightly before serving.

Nutrient	Amount
Calories	400 kcal
Protein	30g
Total Carbohydrates	45g
- Sugars	3g
- Dietary Fiber	6g
Total Fat	15g
- Saturated Fat	3g

Meal Prepping:

Storage: Store the tuna mixture in an airtight container in the refrigerator for up to 2 days. Store the tortilla and vegetables separately to maintain freshness.

Serving: Lay the tortilla flat and arrange the tuna mixture and vegetables in the center, then roll up the tortilla tightly before serving.

Shrimp & Veggie Stir-Fry

Preparation Time: 10 minutes
Cooking Time: 10 minutes
Servings: 1

Ingredients:
- 6 oz Shrimp, peeled and deveined
- 1 cup Mixed Vegetables (e.g. bell peppers, snap peas), sliced
- 1 tbsp Olive Oil
- 1 tbsp Soy Sauce (low sodium)
- 1 tsp Ginger, grated
- 1 Garlic Clove, minced

Instructions: In a skillet, heat olive oil over medium heat. Add shrimp and cook until pink. Add mixed vegetables, soy sauce, ginger, and garlic. Stir-fry until vegetables are tender.

Nutrient	Amount
Calories	350 kcal
Protein	35g
Total Carbohydrates	25g
- Sugars	4g
- Dietary Fiber	5g
Total Fat	15g
- Saturated Fat	2g

Meal Prepping:

Storage: Store the stir-fry in an airtight container in the refrigerator for up to 2 days.
Serving: Reheat in a skillet over medium heat, stirring occasionally, until warmed through.

Turkey & Veggie Bowl

Preparation Time: 10 minutes
Cooking Time: 15 minutes
Servings: 1

Ingredients:
6 oz Ground Turkey
1 cup Mixed Vegetables (e.g. bell peppers, broccoli), diced
½ cup Brown Rice, cooked
1 tbsp Olive Oil
Salt and Pepper, to taste
1 tbsp Salsa

Instructions: In a skillet, heat olive oil over medium heat. Add ground turkey and cook until browned. Add mixed vegetables and sauté until tender. Mix in cooked brown rice, salt, pepper, and salsa before serving.

Nutrient	Amount
Calories	400 kcal
Protein	35g
Total Carbohydrates	45g
- Sugars	4g
- Dietary Fiber	6g
Total Fat	15g
- Saturated Fat	3g

Meal Prepping:
Storage: Store in an airtight container in the refrigerator for up to 3-4 days.
Serving: Reheat in the microwave or in a skillet over medium heat until warmed through.

Salmon & Veggie Pasta

Preparation Time: 10 minutes
Cooking Time: 20 minutes
Servings: 1

Ingredients:
6 oz Salmon Fillet
1 cup Whole Wheat Pasta, cooked
1 cup Mixed Vegetables (e.g. cherry tomatoes, spinach)
1 tbsp Olive Oil
Salt and Pepper, to taste
1 Lemon Slice

Instructions: Preheat oven to 400°F (200°C).
Place salmon on a baking sheet and drizzle with olive oil.
Season with salt and pepper and bake for 20 minutes or until salmon is cooked through.
In a bowl, mix cooked pasta, mixed vegetables, and baked salmon.
Serve with a lemon slice.

Nutrient	Amount
Calories	450 kcal
Protein	35g
Total Carbohydrates	45g
- Sugars	4g
- Dietary Fiber	6g
Total Fat	20g
- Saturated Fat	4g

Meal Prepping:
Storage: Store in an airtight container in the refrigerator for up to 2-3 days.
Serving: Reheat in the microwave or in a skillet over medium heat, adding a little water or broth if needed to prevent dryness.

Chicken & Veggie Skewers

Preparation Time: 10 minutes
Cooking Time: 15 minutes
Servings: 1

Ingredients:
6 oz Chicken Breast, cut into chunks
1 cup Mixed Vegetables (e.g. bell peppers, zucchini), cut into chunks
1 tbsp Olive Oil
Salt and Pepper, to taste
1 Lemon Slice

Instructions: Preheat grill to medium heat.
Thread chicken and vegetable chunks onto skewers.
Drizzle with olive oil and season with salt and pepper.
Grill until chicken is cooked through, turning occasionally.
Serve with a lemon slice.

Nutrient	Amount
Calories	350 kcal
Protein	40g
Total Carbohydrates	15g
- Sugars	3g
- Dietary Fiber	4g
Total Fat	15g
- Saturated Fat	3g

Meal Prepping:
Storage: Store in an airtight container in the refrigerator for up to 3-4 days.
Serving: Reheat on a baking sheet in the oven at 350°F (175°C) for about 10 minutes or until heated through.

6 Nutrient-Dense Suppers

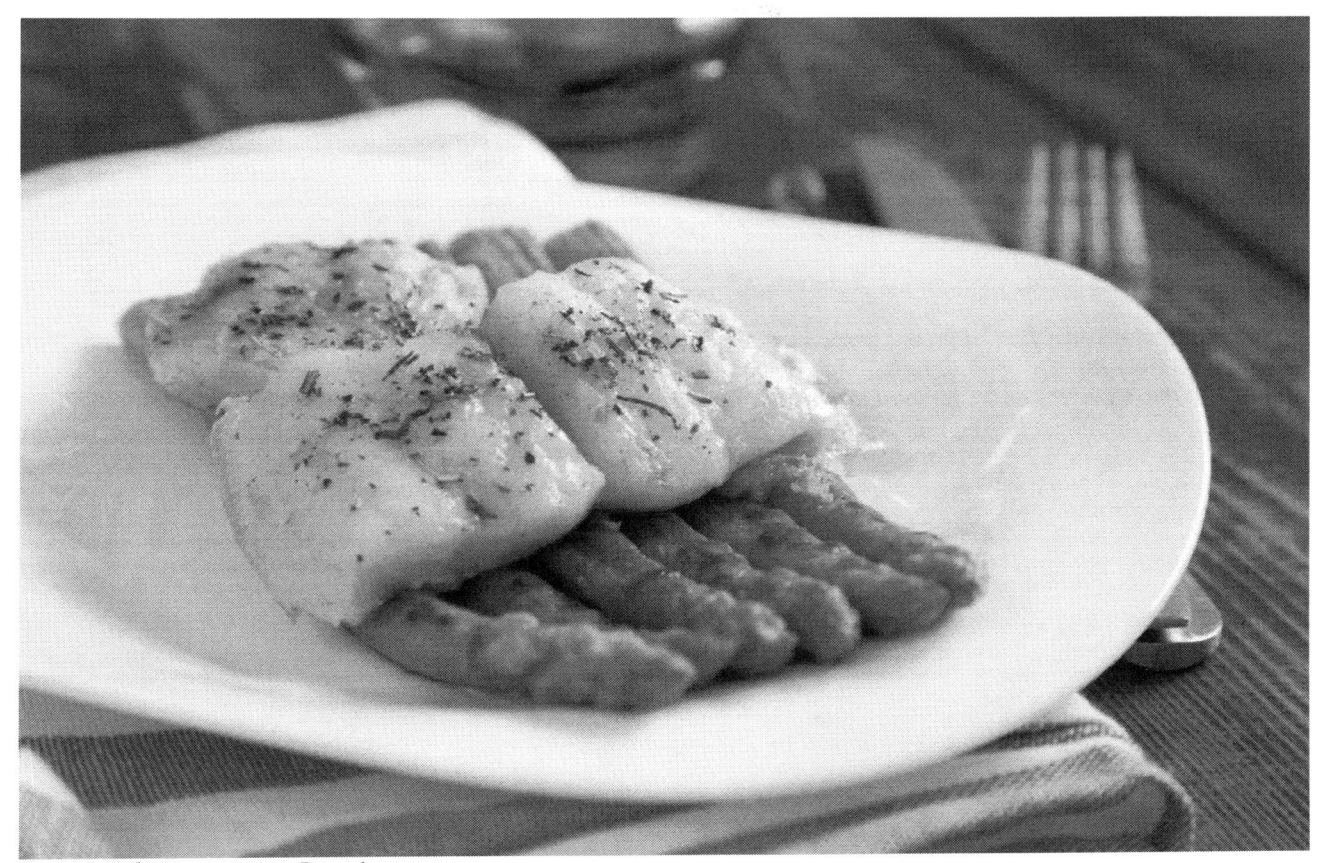

Baked Cod & Asparagus - Page 65

Dinner in bodybuilding meal prep is a strategic meal that plays a pivotal role in recovery and growth as it follows the day's most intense physical exertions. It's designed not only to replenish nutrients lost during workouts but also to facilitate muscle repair, growth, and overall body recuperation overnight. The focus is on proteins, healthy fats, and fibers, with a careful approach to carbohydrates.

These dinner recipes are crafted to ensure that the bodybuilder's nutritional needs are met, even as the body rests. The goal is to wake up recovered, refueled, and ready for another day of pushing physical boundaries.

Please note: the recipes are designed for one serving, allowing you the freedom to determine the number of meals you prepare in advance. Ensure you examine the food's condition before reheating and discard anything that appears or smells suspicious.

Baked Salmon & Steamed Veggies

Preparation Time: 5 minutes

Cooking Time: 20 minutes

Servings: 1

Ingredients:

6 oz Salmon Fillet

1 cup Mixed Vegetables (e.g. broccoli, carrots)

1 tbsp Olive Oil

Salt and Pepper, to taste

1 Lemon Slice

Instructions: Preheat oven to 400°F (200°C).

Place salmon on a baking sheet, drizzle with olive oil, season with salt and pepper.

Bake for 20 minutes or until salmon is cooked through.

Steam mixed vegetables and serve with baked salmon and a lemon slice.

Nutrient	Amount
Calories	450 kcal
Protein	35g
Total Carbohydrates	25g
- Sugars	5g
- Dietary Fiber	5g
Total Fat	20g
- Saturated Fat	3g

Meal Prepping:

Storage: Store in an airtight container in the refrigerator for up to 2-3 days.

Serving: Reheat in the oven at 275°F (135°C) for 10-15 minutes or until warmed through.

Beef Stir-Fry & Brown Rice

Preparation Time: 10 minutes

Cooking Time: 15 minutes

Servings: 1

Ingredients:
6 oz Lean Beef Strips
1 cup Mixed Vegetables (e.g. bell peppers, snap peas)
½ cup Brown Rice, cooked
1 tbsp Olive Oil
1 tbsp Soy Sauce (low sodium)
1 tsp Ginger, grated
1 Garlic Clove, minced

Instructions: In a skillet, heat olive oil over medium heat. Add beef strips and cook until browned. Add mixed vegetables, soy sauce, ginger, and garlic. Stir-fry until vegetables are tender. Serve with cooked brown rice.

Nutrient	Amount
Calories	500 kcal
Protein	35g
Total Carbohydrates	45g
- Sugars	4g
- Dietary Fiber	5g
Total Fat	20g
- Saturated Fat	5g

Meal Prepping:

Storage: Store in an airtight container in the refrigerator for up to 3-4 days.

Serving: Reheat in a skillet over medium heat, stirring occasionally, or in the microwave.

Spaghetti Squash & Turkey Meatballs

Preparation Time: 15 minutes

Cooking Time: 45 minutes

Servings: 1

Ingredients:
- 1 cup Spaghetti Squash, cooked
- 6 oz Ground Turkey
- ½ cup Tomato Sauce (no sugar added)
- 1 tbsp Olive Oil
- Salt and Pepper, to taste
- 1 tbsp Parmesan Cheese, grated

Instructions: Form turkey into small meatballs and bake until fully cooked. Heat tomato sauce in a pan, add cooked meatballs. Serve over cooked spaghetti squash, drizzle with olive oil, season with salt, pepper, and top with parmesan cheese.

Nutrient	Amount
Calories	400 kcal
Protein	35g
Total Carbohydrates	25g
- Sugars	6g
- Dietary Fiber	5g
Total Fat	20g
- Saturated Fat	5g

Meal Prepping:

Storage: Store in an airtight container in the refrigerator for up to 3-4 days.

Serving: Reheat in the microwave, covered, or in a covered skillet over medium heat.

Baked Cod & Asparagus

Preparation Time: 5 minutes
Cooking Time: 20 minutes
Servings: 1

Ingredients:
6 oz Cod Fillet
1 cup Asparagus, trimmed
1 tbsp Olive Oil
Salt and Pepper, to taste
1 Lemon Slice

Instructions: Preheat oven to 400°F (200°C).

Place cod and asparagus on a baking sheet, drizzle with olive oil, season with salt and pepper.

Bake for 20 minutes or until cod is cooked through and asparagus is tender.

Serve with a lemon slice.

Nutrient	Amount
Calories	300 kcal
Protein	35g
Total Carbohydrates	15g
- Sugars	3g
- Dietary Fiber	3g
Total Fat	15g
- Saturated Fat	2g

Meal Prepping:

Storage: Store in an airtight container in the refrigerator for up to 2 days.

Serving: Reheat in the oven at 275°F (135°C) for 10-15 minutes or until warmed through.

Chicken & Vegetable Curry

Preparation Time: 10 minutes
Cooking Time: 20 minutes
Servings: 1

Ingredients:
6 oz Chicken Breast, diced
1 cup Mixed Vegetables (e.g. bell peppers, carrots), diced
½ cup Coconut Milk
1 tbsp Curry Powder
1 tbsp Olive Oil
Salt and Pepper, to taste

Instructions: In a skillet, heat olive oil over medium heat. Add chicken and cook until browned. Add mixed vegetables, curry powder, coconut milk, salt, and pepper. Simmer until vegetables are tender and chicken is cooked through.

Nutrient	Amount
Calories	450 kcal
Protein	35g
Total Carbohydrates	25g
- Sugars	6g
- Dietary Fiber	5g
Total Fat	25g
- Saturated Fat	12g

Meal Prepping:
<u>Storage:</u> Store in an airtight container in the refrigerator for up to 3-4 days.
<u>Serving:</u> Reheat on the stove over medium heat, stirring occasionally, or in the microwave.

Turkey & Sweet Potato Hash

Preparation Time: 10 minutes

Cooking Time: 20 minutes

Servings: 1

Ingredients:
6 oz Ground Turkey
1 medium Sweet Potato, diced
1 tbsp Olive Oil
Salt and Pepper, to taste
1 tsp Paprika

Instructions: In a skillet, heat olive oil over medium heat. Add ground turkey and cook until browned. Add sweet potato and cook until tender. Season with salt, pepper, and paprika before serving.

Nutrient	Amount
Calories	400 kcal
Protein	35g
Total Carbohydrates	35g
- Sugars	7g
- Dietary Fiber	5g
Total Fat	15g
- Saturated Fat	3g

Meal Prepping:

Storage: Store in an airtight container in the refrigerator for up to 3-4 days.

Serving: Reheat in a skillet over medium heat, stirring occasionally, until warmed through.

Salmon with Asparagus and Brown Rice

Preparation Time: 10 minutes

Cooking Time: 20 minutes

Servings: 1

Ingredients:
6 oz salmon fillet
1/2 cup brown rice
6-8 asparagus spears
1 tsp olive oil
Lemon zest, salt, and pepper to taste

Instructions: Season the salmon with lemon zest, salt, and pepper. Grill the salmon until fully cooked. Cook the brown rice as per package instructions. Sauté the asparagus in olive oil until tender. Serve the salmon with asparagus and brown rice.

Nutrient	Amount
Calories	510 kcal
Protein	35g
Total Carbohydrates	50g
- Sugars	3g
- Dietary Fiber	4g
Total Fat	18g
- Saturated Fat	3g

Meal Prepping:

Storage: Store in an airtight container in the refrigerator for up to 2-3 days.

Serving: Reheat in the microwave, covered, stirring the rice and fluffing it with a fork.

Vegetable & Quinoa Stuffed Peppers

Preparation Time: 15 minutes
Cooking Time: 30 minutes
Servings: 1

Ingredients:
1 large Bell Pepper
½ cup Quinoa, cooked
1 cup Mixed Vegetables (e.g. tomatoes, corn), diced
1 tbsp Olive Oil
Salt and Pepper, to taste
1 tbsp Feta Cheese, crumbled

Instructions: Preheat oven to 375°F (190°C).
Cut the top off the bell pepper and remove seeds.
In a bowl, mix quinoa, mixed vegetables, olive oil, salt, and pepper.
Stuff bell pepper with quinoa mixture and bake for 30 minutes or until pepper is tender.
Top with feta cheese before serving.

Nutrient	Amount
Calories	350 kcal
Protein	15g
Total Carbohydrates	45g
- Sugars	5g
- Dietary Fiber	6g
Total Fat	15g
- Saturated Fat	3g

Meal Prepping:
Storage: Wrap tightly in aluminum foil. Store in an airtight container in the refrigerator for up to 3-5 days or freeze for up to 3 months.
Serving: If refrigerated, reheat in the microwave high for 2-3 minutes.
If frozen, thaw in the refrigerator overnight before reheating.

Pork Chop with Green Beans and Almonds

Preparation Time: 10 minutes

Cooking Time: 20 minutes

Servings: 1

Ingredients:

6 oz pork chop

1 cup green beans

10 almonds, chopped

1 tsp olive oil

Salt, pepper, and garlic powder to taste

Instructions: Season the pork chop with salt, pepper, and garlic powder.

Grill or pan-sear the pork chop until fully cooked.

Sauté the green beans in olive oil until tender. Add the chopped almonds and cook for an additional 2 minutes.

Serve the pork chop with the green beans and almonds.

Nutrient	Amount
Calories	500 kcal
Protein	38g
Total Carbohydrates	15g
- Sugars	4g
- Dietary Fiber	4g
Total Fat	30g
- Saturated Fat	8g

Meal Prepping:

Storage: Store the pork chop and green beans in separate airtight containers to prevent the green beans from getting soggy. Refrigerate for up to 3-4 days.

Serving: Reheat the pork chop in the oven at 350°F (175°C) for about 10-15 minutes. Warm the green beans in the microwave for 12 minutes.

Shrimp and Broccoli Stir-Fry

Preparation Time: 10 minutes
Cooking Time: 15 minutes
Servings: 1

Ingredients:
6 oz shrimp, peeled and deveined
1 cup broccoli florets
1 tbsp soy sauce (low sodium)
1 tsp olive oil
1 garlic clove, minced
Red pepper flakes to taste

Instructions: In a pan, heat the olive oil and sauté the garlic until fragrant.

Add the shrimp and cook until pink.

Add the broccoli florets and soy sauce. Cook until the broccoli is tender.

Sprinkle with red pepper flakes for some heat (optional).

Serve hot.

Nutrient	Amount
Calories	320 kcal
Protein	35g
Total Carbohydrates	15g
- Sugars	3g
- Dietary Fiber	4g
Total Fat	12g
- Saturated Fat	2g

Meal Prepping:

Storage: Store in an airtight container in the refrigerator for up to 2 days.

Serving: Reheat in a skillet over medium heat for 5-7 minutes or in the microwave for 2-3 minutes.

Spaghetti Squash & Chicken Parmesan

Preparation Time: 15 minutes
Cooking Time: 45 minutes
Servings: 1

Ingredients:
1 cup Spaghetti Squash, cooked
6 oz Chicken Breast
½ cup Tomato Sauce (no sugar added)
1 tbsp Olive Oil
Salt and Pepper, to taste
1 tbsp Parmesan Cheese, grated

Instructions: Bake chicken until fully cooked. Heat tomato sauce in a pan, add baked chicken. Serve over cooked spaghetti squash, drizzle with olive oil, season with salt, pepper, and top with parmesan cheese.

Nutrient	Amount
Calories	400 kcal
Protein	35g
Total Carbohydrates	25g
- Sugars	6g
- Dietary Fiber	5g
Total Fat	20g
- Saturated Fat	5g

Meal Prepping:

<u>Storage:</u> Store in an airtight container in the refrigerator for up to 3-4 days.

<u>Serving:</u> Reheat in the microwave for 2-3 minutes or in the oven at 350°F (175°C) until hot.

Chicken & Sweet Potato Curry

Preparation Time: 10 minutes
Cooking Time: 20 minutes
Servings: 1

Ingredients:
6 oz Chicken Breast, diced
1 medium Sweet Potato, diced
½ cup Coconut Milk
1 tbsp Curry Powder
1 tbsp Olive Oil
Salt and Pepper, to taste

Instructions: In a skillet, heat olive oil over medium heat.
Add chicken and cook until browned.
Add sweet potato, curry powder, coconut milk, salt, and pepper.
Simmer until sweet potato is tender and chicken is cooked through.

Nutrient	Amount
Calories	450 kcal
Protein	35g
Total Carbohydrates	35g
- Sugars	7g
- Dietary Fiber	5g
Total Fat	25g
- Saturated Fat	12g

Meal Prepping:

Storage: Store in an airtight container in the refrigerator for up to 3-4 days.

Serving: Reheat on the stove over medium heat or in the microwave until warmed through.

Shrimp & Cauliflower Rice

Preparation Time: 10 minutes
Cooking Time: 10 minutes
Servings: 1

Ingredients:
6 oz Shrimp, peeled and deveined
1 cup Cauliflower Rice
1 tbsp Olive Oil
1 Garlic Clove, minced
Salt and Pepper, to taste
1 tbsp Parmesan Cheese, grated

Instructions: In a skillet, heat olive oil over medium heat.
Add shrimp and cook until pink.
Add cauliflower rice, garlic, salt, and pepper.
Sauté until rice is tender.
Top with parmesan cheese before serving.

Nutrient	Amount
Calories	350 kcal
Protein	35g
Total Carbohydrates	15g
- Sugars	3g
- Dietary Fiber	5g
Total Fat	20g
- Saturated Fat	3g

Meal Prepping:
Storage: Store in an airtight container in the refrigerator for up to 2 days.
Serving: Reheat in a skillet over medium heat or in the microwave for 2-3 minutes.

Turkey & Butternut Squash Hash

Preparation Time: 10 minutes

Cooking Time: 20 minutes

Servings: 1

Ingredients:

6 oz Ground Turkey

1 cup Butternut Squash, diced

1 tbsp Olive Oil

Salt and Pepper, to taste

1 tsp Cinnamon

Instructions: In a skillet, heat olive oil over medium heat. Add ground turkey and cook until browned. Add butternut squash and cook until tender. Season with salt, pepper, and cinnamon before serving.

Nutrient	Amount
Calories	400 kcal
Protein	35g
Total Carbohydrates	35g
- Sugars	5g
- Dietary Fiber	6g
Total Fat	15g
- Saturated Fat	3g

Meal Prepping:

Storage: Store in an airtight container in the refrigerator for up to 3-4 days.

Serving: Reheat in a skillet over medium heat, stirring occasionally, or in the microwave.

Vegetable & Farro Stuffed Tomatoes

Preparation Time: 15 minutes

Cooking Time: 30 minutes

Servings: 1

Ingredients:
- 1 large Tomato
- ½ cup Farro, cooked
- 1 cup Mixed Vegetables (e.g. zucchini, corn), diced
- 1 tbsp Olive Oil
- Salt and Pepper, to taste
- 1 tbsp Goat Cheese, crumbled

Instructions: Preheat oven to 375°F (190°C).

Cut the top off the tomato and remove seeds.

In a bowl, mix farro, mixed vegetables, olive oil, salt, and pepper.

Stuff tomato with farro mixture and bake for 30 minutes or until tomato is tender.

Top with goat cheese before serving.

Nutrient	Amount
Calories	350 kcal
Protein	15g
Total Carbohydrates	45g
- Sugars	5g
- Dietary Fiber	8g
Total Fat	15g
- Saturated Fat	3g

Meal Prepping:

Storage: Store in an airtight container for up to 3 days.

Serving: Reheat in the oven at 350°F (175°C) for 10-15 minutes.

Baked Tilapia & Green Beans

Preparation Time: 5 minutes

Cooking Time: 20 minutes

Servings: 1

Ingredients:
6 oz Tilapia Fillet
1 cup Green Beans, trimmed
1 tbsp Olive Oil
Salt and Pepper, to taste
1 Lemon Slice

Instructions: Preheat oven to 400°F (200°C).

Place tilapia and green beans on a baking sheet, drizzle with olive oil, season with salt and pepper.

Bake for 20 minutes or until tilapia is cooked through and green beans are tender.

Serve with a lemon slice.

Nutrient	Amount
Calories	300 kcal
Protein	35g
Total Carbohydrates	15g
- Sugars	3g
- Dietary Fiber	4g
Total Fat	15g
- Saturated Fat	3g

Meal Prepping:

<u>Storage:</u> Store Store in an airtight container in the refrigerator for up to 2 days.

<u>Serving:</u> Reheat the tilapia in the oven at 275°F (135°C) for 10-15 minutes and the green beans in the microwave for 1-2 minutes.

Chicken & Mango Salad

Preparation Time: 10 minutes

Cooking Time: 15 minutes

Servings: 1

Ingredients:

6 oz Chicken Breast

1 cup Mixed Greens

½ medium Mango, sliced

1 tbsp Olive Oil

Salt and Pepper, to taste

1 tbsp Balsamic Vinegar

Instructions: Grill chicken until fully cooked.

In a bowl, mix mixed greens, mango, olive oil, salt, pepper, and balsamic vinegar.

Top with grilled chicken.

Nutrient	Amount
Calories	400 kcal
Protein	35g
Total Carbohydrates	25g
- Sugars	20g
- Dietary Fiber	3g
Total Fat	20g
- Saturated Fat	4g

Meal Prepping:

<u>Storage:</u> Store the grilled chicken in an airtight container in the refrigerator for up to 3-4 days.

Keep the mixed greens and mango in separate containers to maintain freshness and add the dressing just before serving.

<u>Serving:</u> Assemble the salad with the greens and mango, top with sliced chicken, and drizzle with the dressing.

Beef & Brussels Sprouts Stir-Fry

Preparation Time: 10 minutes
Cooking Time: 15 minutes
Servings: 1

Ingredients:
6 oz Lean Beef Strips
1 cup Brussels Sprouts, halved
1 tbsp Olive Oil
1 tbsp Soy Sauce (low sodium)
1 tsp Ginger, grated
1 Garlic Clove, minced

Instructions: In a skillet, heat olive oil over medium heat. Add beef strips and cook until browned. Add Brussels sprouts, soy sauce, ginger, and garlic. Stir-fry until Brussels sprouts are tender.

Nutrient	Amount
Calories	400 kcal
Protein	35g
Total Carbohydrates	15g
- Sugars	4g
- Dietary Fiber	4g
Total Fat	25g
- Saturated Fat	8g

Meal Prepping:
Storage: Store in an airtight container in the refrigerator for up to 3-4 days.
Serving: Reheat in a skillet over medium heat for 5-7 minutes, stirring occasionally, or microwave for 2-3 minutes.

Vegetable & Egg Fried Rice

Preparation Time: 5 minutes
Cooking Time: 10 minutes
Servings: 1

Ingredients:
1 cup Mixed Vegetables (e.g. peas, carrots), chopped
1 cup Cauliflower Rice
2 Large Eggs
1 tbsp Olive Oil
Salt and Pepper, to taste
1 tbsp Soy Sauce (low sodium)

Instructions: In a skillet, heat olive oil over medium heat.
Add mixed vegetables and sauté until tender.
Add cauliflower rice and cook until tender.
Push rice to one side of the skillet, crack eggs into the other side, and scramble.
Mix eggs with rice, season with salt, pepper, and soy sauce.

Nutrient	Amount
Calories	350 kcal
Protein	25g
Total Carbohydrates	25g
- Sugars	5g
- Dietary Fiber	6g
Total Fat	20g
- Saturated Fat	4g

Meal Prepping:
<u>Storage:</u> Store the pancakes in an airtight container in the refrigerator for up to 3 days.
<u>Serving:</u> Reheat in a skillet over medium heat or in the microwave for 1-2 minutes, stirring halfway through.

Chicken & Pumpkin Curry

Preparation Time: 10 minutes

Cooking Time: 20 minutes

Servings: 1

Ingredients:

6 oz Chicken Breast, diced

1 cup Pumpkin, diced

½ cup Coconut Milk

1 tbsp Curry Powder

1 tbsp Olive Oil

Salt and Pepper, to taste

Instructions: In a skillet, heat olive oil over medium heat. Add chicken and cook until browned. Add pumpkin, curry powder, coconut milk, salt, and pepper. Simmer until pumpkin is tender and chicken is cooked through.

Nutrient	Amount
Calories	450 kcal
Protein	35g
Total Carbohydrates	25g
- Sugars	6g
- Dietary Fiber	5g
Total Fat	25g
- Saturated Fat	12g

Meal Prepping:

<u>Storage:</u> Store in an airtight container in the refrigerator for up to 3-4 days.

<u>Serving:</u> Reheat on the stove over medium heat, stirring occasionally, or in the microwave until warmed through.

Turkey & Acorn Squash Hash

Preparation Time: 10 minutes

Cooking Time: 20 minutes

Servings: 1

Ingredients:
6 oz Ground Turkey
1 cup Acorn Squash, diced
1 tbsp Olive Oil
Salt and Pepper, to taste
1 tsp Nutmeg

Instructions: In a skillet, heat olive oil over medium heat.
Add ground turkey and cook until browned.
Add acorn squash and cook until tender.
Season with salt, pepper, and nutmeg before serving.

Nutrient	Amount
Calories	400 kcal
Protein	35g
Total Carbohydrates	35g
- Sugars	4g
- Dietary Fiber	6g
Total Fat	15g
- Saturated Fat	4g

Meal Prepping:

Storage: Store in an airtight container for up to 3-4 days.

Serving: Reheat in a skillet over medium heat, stirring occasionally, or in the microwave.

Vegetable & Bulgur Stuffed Eggplant

Preparation Time: 15 minutes
Cooking Time: 30 minutes
Servings: 1

Ingredients:
1 medium Eggplant
½ cup Bulgur, cooked
1 cup Mixed Vegetables (e.g. bell peppers, tomatoes), diced
1 tbsp Olive Oil
Salt and Pepper, to taste
1 tbsp Feta Cheese, crumbled

Instructions: Preheat oven to 375°F (190°C).

Cut the eggplant in half lengthwise and scoop out the flesh.

In a bowl, mix bulgur, mixed vegetables, olive oil, salt, and pepper.

Stuff eggplant halves with bulgur mixture and bake for 30 minutes or until eggplant is tender.

Top with feta cheese before serving.

Nutrient	Amount
Calories	350 kcal
Protein	15g
Total Carbohydrates	45g
- Sugars	6g
- Dietary Fiber	10g
Total Fat	15g
- Saturated Fat	3g

Meal Prepping:

Storage: Store in an airtight container for up to 3 days.

Serving: Reheat in the oven at 350°F (175°C) for 10-15 minutes.

Baked Haddock & Roasted Vegetables

Preparation Time: 5 minutes
Cooking Time: 20 minutes
Servings: 1

Ingredients:
6 oz Haddock Fillet
1 cup Mixed Vegetables (e.g. bell peppers, zucchini), diced
1 tbsp Olive Oil
Salt and Pepper, to taste
1 Lemon Slice

Instructions: Preheat oven to 400°F (200°C).

Place haddock and mixed vegetables on a baking sheet, drizzle with olive oil, season with salt and pepper.

Bake for 20 minutes or until haddock is cooked through and vegetables are tender.

Serve with a lemon slice.

Nutrient	Amount
Calories	300 kcal
Protein	35g
Total Carbohydrates	25g
- Sugars	5g
- Dietary Fiber	6g
Total Fat	15g
- Saturated Fat	3g

Meal Prepping:

Storage: Store in an airtight container in the refrigerator for up to 2-3 days.

Serving: Reheat the haddock in the oven at 275°F (135°C) for 10-15 minutes and the vegetables in the microwave for 1-2 minutes.

Chicken & Pineapple Salad

Preparation Time: 10 minutes
Cooking Time: 15 minutes
Servings: 1

Ingredients:
6 oz Chicken Breast
1 cup Mixed Greens
½ cup Pineapple, diced
1 tbsp Olive Oil
Salt and Pepper, to taste
1 tbsp Balsamic Vinegar

Instructions: Grill chicken until fully cooked.
In a bowl, mix mixed greens, pineapple, olive oil, salt, pepper, and balsamic vinegar.
Top with grilled chicken.

Nutrient	Amount
Calories	400 kcal
Protein	35g
Total Carbohydrates	35g
- Sugars	20g
- Dietary Fiber	3g
Total Fat	20g
- Saturated Fat	4g

Meal Prepping:

<u>Storage:</u> Store the grilled chicken in an airtight container in the refrigerator for up to 3-4 days.
Keep the mixed greens and pineapple in separate containers to maintain freshness and add the dressing just before serving.
<u>Serving:</u> Assemble the salad with the greens and pineapple, top with sliced chicken, and drizzle with the dressing.

Beef & Cabbage Stir-Fry

Preparation Time: 10 minutes
Cooking Time: 15 minutes
Servings: 1

Ingredients:
6 oz Lean Beef Strips
1 cup Cabbage, shredded
1 tbsp Olive Oil
1 tbsp Soy Sauce (low sodium)
1 tsp Ginger, grated
1 Garlic Clove, minced

Instructions: In a skillet, heat olive oil over medium heat. Add beef strips and cook until browned. Add cabbage, soy sauce, ginger, and garlic. Stir-fry until cabbage is tender.

Nutrient	Amount
Calories	400 kcal
Protein	35g
Total Carbohydrates	15g
- Sugars	4g
- Dietary Fiber	4g
Total Fat	25g
- Saturated Fat	8g

Meal Prepping:
Storage: Store in an airtight container in the refrigerator for up to 3-4 days.
Serving: Reheat in a skillet over medium heat for 5-7 minutes or in the microwave for 2-3 minutes.

7 Smart Snack Choices

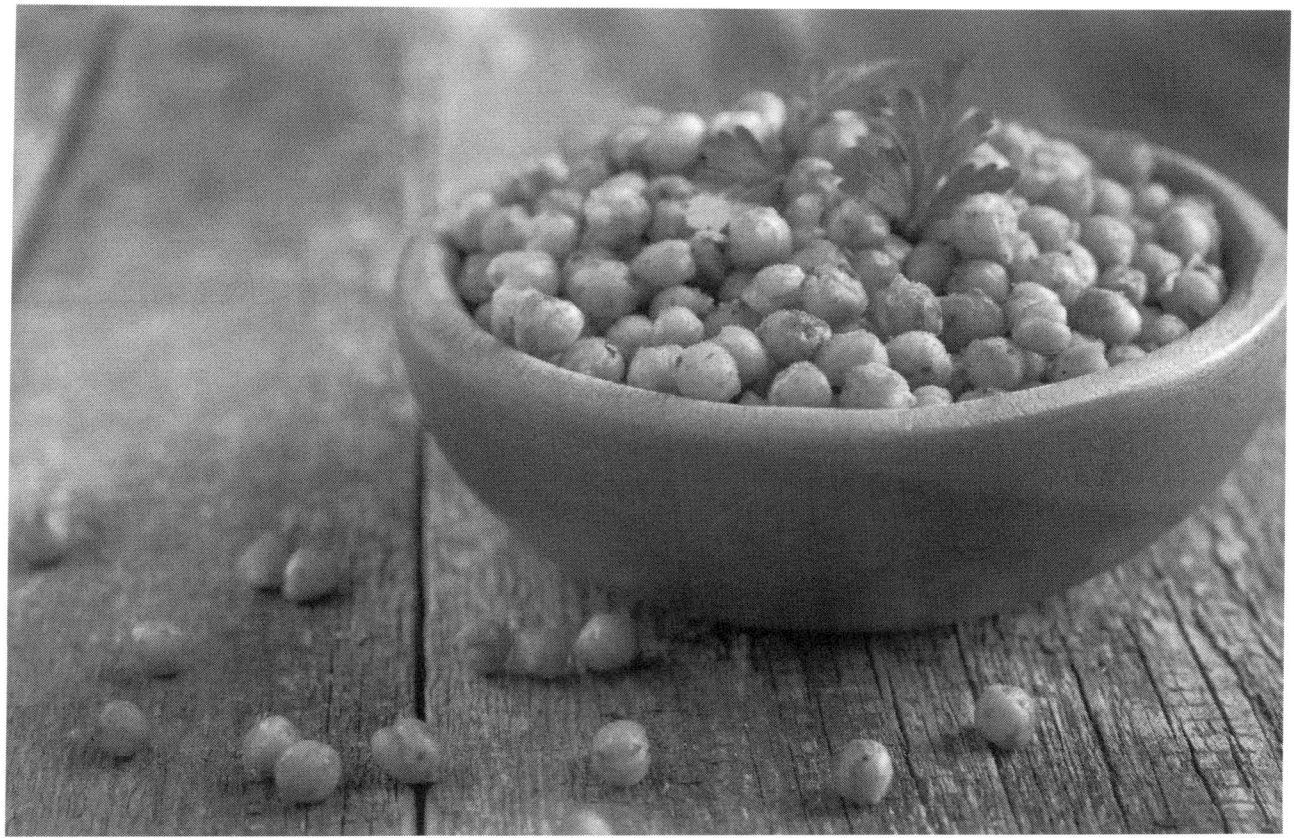

Spicy Roasted Chickpeas - Page 91

Snacks in bodybuilding meal prep serve crucial roles: they keep energy levels steady between meals, aid in maintaining an anabolic state, and ensure the body is fueled for recovery and growth throughout the day. These mini-meals are meticulously crafted to provide a balanced blend of proteins, healthy fats, and carbohydrates, catering to immediate energy needs while contributing to longer-term muscle repair and building.

Snack recipes in bodybuilding are far from arbitrary; they're strategic, delicious fueling sessions that work in concert with main meals to support an athlete's rigorous training regimen and physique goals. They're convenient, portable, and designed to satiate hunger while providing substantial nutritional value.

Please note: the recipes are designed for one serving, allowing you the freedom to determine the number of meals you prepare in advance. Ensure you examine the food's condition before reheating and discard anything that appears or smells suspicious.

Power Protein Balls

Preparation Time: 10 minutes

Cooking Time: 0 minutes

Servings: 1

Ingredients:

2 tbsp natural peanut butter

1 scoop whey protein powder (chocolate or vanilla)

1 tbsp honey

1 tbsp rolled oats

1 tsp chia seeds.

Instructions: Mix all ingredients in a bowl until well combined.

Roll into bite-sized balls.

Refrigerate for 30 minutes before serving.

Nutrient	Amount
Calories	310 kcal
Protein	20g
Total Carbohydrates	25g
- Sugars	12g
- Dietary Fiber	3g
Total Fat	15g
- Saturated Fat	3g

Meal Prepping:

Storage: Store the protein balls in an airtight container in the refrigerator for up to 7 days.

Serving: Serve chilled.

Quinoa & Vegetable Salad

Preparation Time: 10 minutes
Cooking Time: 15 minutes
Servings: 1

Ingredients:
½ cup Quinoa, cooked
1 cup Mixed Vegetables (e.g. cucumber, cherry tomatoes), diced
1 tbsp Olive Oil
Salt and Pepper, to taste
1 tbsp Lemon Juice

Instructions: Mix quinoa, mixed vegetables, olive oil, salt, pepper, and lemon juice. Serve chilled or at room temperature.

Nutrient	Amount
Calories	250 kcal
Protein	10g
Total Carbohydrates	35g
- Sugars	5g
- Dietary Fiber	5g
Total Fat	15g
- Saturated Fat	2g

Meal Prepping:
Storage: Store the salad in an airtight container in the refrigerator for up to 3-5 days.
Serving: Serve chilled or at room temperature. Toss before serving if ingredients have settled.

Nutty Protein Bars

Preparation Time: 15 minutes
Cooking Time: 0 minutes (Chill for 1 hour)
Servings: 1

Ingredients:
- 1 scoop Protein powder (vanilla)
- 2 tbsp Rolled oats
- 1 tbsp Natural peanut butter
- 1 tbsp Almonds (chopped)
- 1 tsp Honey
- 1 tbsp Dark chocolate chips

Instructions: In a bowl, mix all ingredients until well combined. Press the mixture into a small container or mold. Chill in the refrigerator for 1 hour before cutting into bars.

Nutrient	Amount
Calories	320 kcal
Protein	20g
Total Carbohydrates	30g
- Sugars	10g
- Dietary Fiber	4g
Total Fat	15g
- Saturated Fat	3g

Meal Prepping:

Storage: After chilling and cutting into bars, store them in an airtight container in the refrigerator for up to 7 days or freeze for up to 1 month.

Serving: Enjoy chilled as a quick snack or post-workout protein boost.

Spicy Roasted Chickpeas

Preparation Time: 5 minutes

Cooking Time: 30 minutes

Servings: 1

Ingredients:

1 cup Chickpeas, drained and rinsed

1 tbsp Olive Oil

1 tsp Paprika

Salt and Pepper, to taste

Instructions: Preheat oven to 400°F (200°C).

Toss chickpeas with olive oil, paprika, salt, and pepper.

Spread on a baking sheet and roast for 30 minutes or until crispy.

Nutrient	Amount
Calories	300 kcal
Protein	15g
Total Carbohydrates	35g
- Sugars	6g
- Dietary Fiber	9g
Total Fat	15g
- Saturated Fat	2g

Meal Prepping:

Storage: Store them in an airtight container at room temperature for up to 7 days.

Serving: Enjoy as a crunchy snack on their own or as a topping for salads.

Baked Sweet Potato Fries

Preparation Time: 10 minutes

Cooking Time: 30 minutes

Servings: 1

Ingredients:
1 medium Sweet Potato, sliced into fries
1 tbsp Olive Oil
Salt and Pepper, to taste
1 tsp Cinnamon

Instructions: Preheat oven to 400°F (200°C).

Toss sweet potato fries with olive oil, salt, pepper, and cinnamon.

Spread on a baking sheet and bake for 30 minutes or until crispy.

Nutrient	Amount
Calories	200 kcal
Protein	3g
Total Carbohydrates	35g
- Sugars	7g
- Dietary Fiber	5g
Total Fat	7g
- Saturated Fat	1g

Meal Prepping:

Storage: Store the fries in an airtight container in the refrigerator for up to 3 days.

Serving: Reheat in the oven at 400°F (200°C) for 5-10 minutes or until crispy again.

Protein-Packed Trail Mix

Preparation Time: 5 minutes
Cooking Time: 0 minutes
Servings: 1

Ingredients:
2 tbsp almonds
1 tbsp walnuts
1 tbsp dried cranberries
1 tbsp pumpkin seeds.

Instructions: Mix all ingredients in a small bag or bowl. Enjoy as a quick snack.

Nutrient	Amount
Calories	250 kcal
Protein	8g
Total Carbohydrates	15g
- Sugars	7g
- Dietary Fiber	4g
Total Fat	18g
- Saturated Fat	2g

Meal Prepping:

Storage: Store the trail mix in an airtight container or a ziplock bag to prevent it from getting stale. It can be stored at room temperature for up to 1 month.

Serving: Serve as is. No reheating is necessary.

Spicy Mixed Nuts

Preparation Time: 5 minutes
Cooking Time: 10 minutes
Servings: 1

Ingredients:
1 cup Mixed Nuts (e.g. almonds, walnuts)
1 tbsp Olive Oil
1 tsp Cayenne Pepper
Salt, to taste

Instructions: Preheat oven to 350°F (180°C).

Toss mixed nuts with olive oil, cayenne pepper, and salt.

Spread on a baking sheet and roast for 10 minutes or until golden.

Nutrient	Amount
Calories	400 kcal
Protein	10g
Total Carbohydrates	15g
- Sugars	4g
- Dietary Fiber	4g
Total Fat	35g
- Saturated Fat	5g

Meal Prepping:

Storage: Store them in an airtight container at room temperature for up to 14 days.

Serving: Enjoy as a savory snack on their own.

Berry & Oat Protein Bars

Preparation Time: 10 minutes
Cooking Time: 20 minutes
Servings: 1

Ingredients:
½ cup Rolled Oats
1 scoop Protein Powder
½ cup Mixed Berries (e.g. raspberries, blueberries)
1 tbsp Honey
1 tbsp Almond Butter

Instructions: Preheat oven to 350°F (180°C).
Mix rolled oats, protein powder, mixed berries, honey, and almond butter.
Press into a small baking dish and bake for 20 minutes or until golden.
Cool and cut into bars.

Nutrient	Amount
Calories	350 kcal
Protein	25g
Total Carbohydrates	45g
- Sugars	15g
- Dietary Fiber	5g
Total Fat	10g
- Saturated Fat	2g

Meal Prepping:
Storage: After baking and cutting into bars, store them in an airtight container in the refrigerator for up to 7 days or freeze for up to 2 months.
Serving: These can be enjoyed cold or brought to room temperature for a softer texture.

Veggie & Quinoa Bites

Preparation Time: 10 minutes
Cooking Time: 20 minutes
Servings: 1

Ingredients:
½ cup Quinoa, cooked
1 cup Mixed Vegetables (e.g. carrots, bell peppers), finely diced
1 Egg
Salt and Pepper, to taste
1 tbsp Parmesan Cheese, grated

Instructions: Preheat oven to 375°F (190°C).

Mix quinoa, mixed vegetables, egg, salt, pepper, and parmesan cheese.

Spoon into mini muffin tins and bake for 20 minutes or until golden.

Nutrient	Amount
Calories	300 kcal
Protein	15g
Total Carbohydrates	35g
- Sugars	4g
- Dietary Fiber	5g
Total Fat	10g
- Saturated Fat	2g

Meal Prepping:

Storage: Store them in an airtight container in the refrigerator for up to 5 days.

Serving: Reheat in a microwave for 30-60 seconds or in an oven at 350°F (175°C) for 5-10 minutes until heated through.

Veggie Sticks with Hummus Dip

Preparation Time: 10 minutes
Cooking Time: 0 minutes
Servings: 1

Ingredients:
Hummus: ¼ cup
Carrot sticks: 5-6
Cucumber sticks: 5-6
Bell pepper strips: 5-6

<u>Homemade Hummus:</u>
- 1 cup canned chickpeas, drained and rinsed
- 1 tbsp tahini
- 1 clove garlic, minced
- Zest and juice of 1 small lemon
- 1 tbsp Olive Oil
- 1 tbsp Mixed Fresh Herbs
- Salt and Pepper to taste
- 1-2 tbsp cold water

Instructions: For the homemade hummus, combine all ingredients in a blender or food processor and blend until smooth. If the mixture is too thick, add cold water, one tablespoon at a time, until you reach the desired consistency.
Serve veggie sticks with a side of hummus for dipping.

Nutrient	Amount
Calories	180 kcal
Protein	6g
Total Carbohydrates	25g
- Sugars	6g
- Dietary Fiber	7g
Total Fat	8g
- Saturated Fat	1g

Meal Prepping:
<u>Storage:</u> Store the cutted veggies in an airtight container or a zip-lock bag with a paper towel to absorb excess moisture. They should last in the refrigerator for 2-3 days.
Store the hummus in a separate airtight container in the refrigerator for up to 7 days.
<u>Serving:</u> Serve the veggie sticks with hummus on the side for dipping. Best enjoyed fresh.

Zucchini & Parmesan Chips

Preparation Time: 10 minutes
Cooking Time: 20 minutes
Servings: 1

Ingredients:
1 medium Zucchini, sliced into thin rounds
1 tbsp Olive Oil
Salt and Pepper, to taste
2 tbsp Parmesan Cheese, grated

Instructions: Preheat oven to 400°F (200°C).
Toss zucchini rounds with olive oil, salt, and pepper.
Arrange on a baking sheet and sprinkle with parmesan cheese.
Bake for 20 minutes or until golden and crispy.

Nutrient	Amount
Calories	200 kcal
Protein	10g
Total Carbohydrates	15g
- Sugars	3g
- Dietary Fiber	2g
Total Fat	15g
- Saturated Fat	4g

Meal Prepping:
Storage: Store the chips in an airtight container at room temperature for up to 2 days. They might lose their crispiness over time.
Serving: Reheat in the oven at 350°F (175°C) for 5-7 minutes to regain crispiness.

8 Post-Workout Refueling Recipes

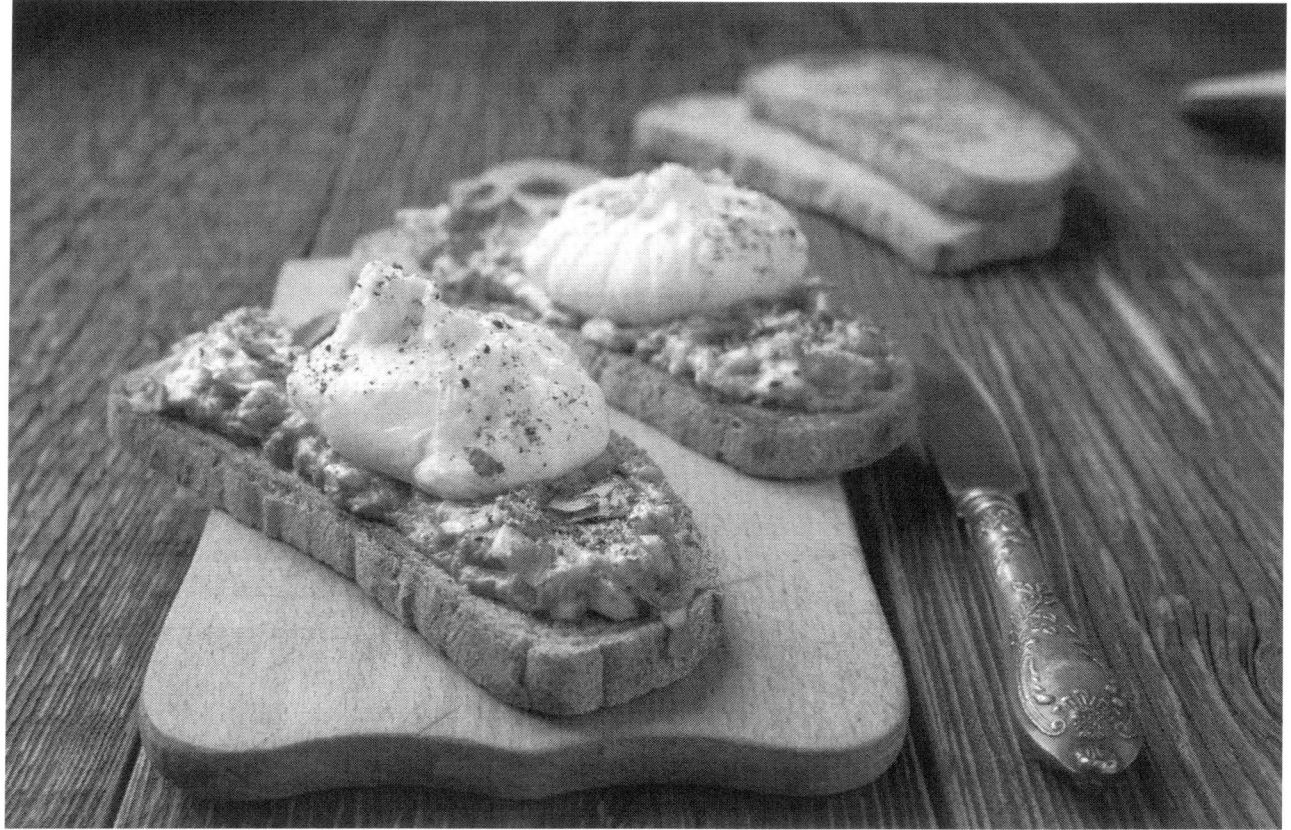

Avocado & Egg Toast - Page 108

Post-workout nutrition in bodybuilding meal prep is a critical component, designed to kickstart the recovery process, replenish energy stores, and support muscle repair and growth after intense training sessions. These meals are scientifically formulated to provide a precise blend of macronutrients, primarily focusing on proteins and carbohydrates, to optimize the body's repair phase.

Post-workout recipes are more than meals; they're part of a holistic strategy to capitalize on the body's anabolic window, facilitating faster recovery, minimizing muscle soreness, and maximizing the muscle-building potential. They're crafted to be appetizing, easy to digest, and quick to prepare, acknowledging that post-workout nutrition is time-sensitive and essential for bodybuilding success.

Please note: the recipes are designed for one serving, allowing you the freedom to determine the number of meals you prepare in advance. Ensure you examine the food's condition before reheating and discard anything that appears or smells suspicious.

Quinoa & Chicken Bowl

Preparation Time: 10 minutes

Cooking Time: 20 minutes

Servings: 1

Ingredients:

1 cup Cooked Quinoa

4 oz Grilled Chicken Breast, sliced

½ cup Cherry Tomatoes, halved

1 tbsp Olive Oil

Salt and Pepper, to taste

Instructions: Mix all ingredients in a bowl. Serve immediately.

Nutrient	Amount
Calories	400 kcal
Protein	35g
Total Carbohydrates	35g
- Sugars	3g
- Dietary Fiber	4g
Total Fat	15g
- Saturated Fat	2.5g

Meal Prepping:

Storage: Store cooked quinoa and grilled chicken separately in airtight containers in the refrigerator for up to 3-4 days.

Serving: Reheat the quinoa and chicken in the microwave for 1-2 minutes or until heated through.

Mix the quinoa, chicken, and fresh cherry tomatoes. Drizzle with olive oil, season, and serve.

Sweet Potato & Turkey Skillet

Preparation Time: 10 minutes

Cooking Time: 20 minutes

Servings: 1

Ingredients:

1 medium Sweet Potato, diced

4 oz Ground Turkey

1 tbsp Olive Oil

Salt and Pepper, to taste

Instructions: In a skillet, heat olive oil and cook sweet potato until tender. Add ground turkey and cook until browned. Season with salt and pepper. Serve immediately.

Nutrient	Amount
Calories	350 kcal
Protein	30g
Total Carbohydrates	30g
- Sugars	6g
- Dietary Fiber	4g
Total Fat	15g
- Saturated Fat	3g

Meal Prepping:

Storage: Store them in an airtight container in the refrigerator for up to 3-4 days.

Serving: Reheat in a skillet over medium heat for 5-7 minutes or microwave for 2-3 minutes.

Salmon & Asparagus Bake

Preparation Time: 10 minutes
Cooking Time: 20 minutes
Servings: 1

Ingredients:
4 oz Salmon Fillet
5 Asparagus Spears
1 tbsp Olive Oil
Lemon Slices
Salt and Pepper, to taste

Instructions: Preheat oven to 400°F (200°C). Place salmon and asparagus on a baking sheet. Drizzle with olive oil and season with salt and pepper. Top with lemon slices and bake for 20 minutes. Serve immediately.

Nutrient	Amount
Calories	300 kcal
Protein	25g
Total Carbohydrates	5g
- Sugars	2g
- Dietary Fiber	2g
Total Fat	20g
- Saturated Fat	3g

Meal Prepping:
Storage: Store in an airtight container in the refrigerator for up to 2 days.
Serving: Reheat in the oven at 275°F (135°C) for 10-15 minutes to maintain the dish's moisture.

Chicken & Avocado Salad

Preparation Time: 10 minutes

Cooking Time: 0 minutes

Servings: 1

Ingredients:
- 4 oz Grilled Chicken Breast, sliced
- 1 medium Avocado, diced
- 2 cups Mixed Greens
- 1 tbsp Olive Oil
- 1 tbsp Balsamic Vinegar
- Salt and Pepper, to taste

Instructions: In a bowl, mix chicken, avocado, and mixed greens. Drizzle with olive oil and balsamic vinegar. Season with salt and pepper. Serve immediately.

Nutrient	Amount
Calories	450 kcal
Protein	35g
Total Carbohydrates	15g
- Sugars	2g
- Dietary Fiber	8g
Total Fat	30g
- Saturated Fat	4.5g

Meal Prepping:

<u>Storage:</u> Store Salad ingredients separately in an airtight container in the refrigerator for up to 2 days.

Best to cut the avocado fresh to prevent browning.

<u>Serving:</u> Combine ingredients, drizzle with the dressing, and serve immediately.

Protein Pancakes

Preparation Time: 10 minutes

Cooking Time: 10 minutes

Servings: 1

Ingredients:

1 scoop Protein Powder

1 medium Banana, mashed

1 large Egg

1 tbsp Almond Milk

Instructions: In a bowl, mix all ingredients until smooth. Cook on a non-stick skillet over medium heat until golden brown on both sides. Serve immediately with your favorite toppings.

Nutrient	Amount
Calories	300 kcal
Protein	30g
Total Carbohydrates	30g
- Sugars	17g
- Dietary Fiber	4g
Total Fat	10g
- Saturated Fat	2g

Meal Prepping:

Storage: Store the pancakes in an airtight container in the refrigerator for up to 2 days or freeze for up to 1 month.

Serving: Reheat in the microwave for 20-30 seconds or in a toaster oven.

Beef & Broccoli Stir-Fry

Preparation Time: 10 minutes

Cooking Time: 15 minutes

Servings: 1

Ingredients:
- 4 oz Lean Beef Strips
- 1 cup Broccoli Florets
- 1 tbsp Soy Sauce
- 1 tbsp Olive Oil
- 1 tsp Sesame Seeds

Instructions: In a skillet, heat olive oil and cook beef until browned. Add broccoli and soy sauce, and stir-fry until broccoli is tender. Sprinkle with sesame seeds and serve immediately.

Nutrient	Amount
Calories	350 kcal
Protein	30g
Total Carbohydrates	10g
- Sugars	2g
- Dietary Fiber	3g
Total Fat	20g
- Saturated Fat	5g

Meal Prepping:

Storage: Store them in an airtight container in the refrigerator for up to 3 days.

Serving: Reheat in a skillet over medium heat for 5 minutes or in the microwave for 1-2 minutes.

Mango & Cottage Cheese Bowl

Preparation Time: 5 minutes

Cooking Time: 0 minutes

Servings: 1

Ingredients:
1 cup Cottage Cheese
½ medium Mango, diced
1 tbsp Honey
1 tbsp Almonds, chopped

Instructions: In a bowl, mix cottage cheese and mango. Drizzle with honey and top with chopped almonds. Serve immediately.

Nutrient	Amount
Calories	300 kcal
Protein	25g
Total Carbohydrates	35g
- Sugars	30g
- Dietary Fiber	3g
Total Fat	10g
- Saturated Fat	2.5g

Meal Prepping:

Storage: Store cottage cheese and mango separately in airtight containers in the refrigerator for up to 2 days. Store chopped almonds at room temperature.

Serving: Mix cottage cheese and mango, drizzle with honey, and sprinkle with almonds just before serving.

Oatmeal & Berry Bowl

Preparation Time: 5 minutes
Cooking Time: 10 minutes
Servings: 1

Ingredients:
½ cup Rolled Oats
1 cup Water
½ cup Mixed Berries
1 tbsp Honey
1 tbsp Chia Seeds

Instructions: Cook oats in water according to package instructions. Top with mixed berries, honey, and chia seeds. Serve immediately.

Nutrient	Amount
Calories	300 kcal
Protein	10g
Total Carbohydrates	50g
- Sugars	20g
- Dietary Fiber	7g
Total Fat	10g
- Saturated Fat	1.5g

Meal Prepping:

Storage: Store in the refrigerator for up to 5 days. Keep berries separately to prevent sogginess.

Serving: Reheat oatmeal in the microwave for 1-2 minutes.

Avocado & Egg Toast

Preparation Time: 5 minutes
Cooking Time: 5 minutes
Servings: 1

Ingredients:
1 slice Whole Grain Bread, toasted
1 medium Avocado, mashed
1 large Egg, poached
Salt and Pepper, to taste

Instructions: Spread mashed avocado on toast. Top with poached egg. Season with salt and pepper. Serve immediately.

Nutrient	Amount
Calories	350 kcal
Protein	12g
Total Carbohydrates	30g
- Sugars	4g
- Dietary Fiber	9g
Total Fat	20g
- Saturated Fat	3.5g

Meal Prepping:

Storage: Store the cooked poached eggs in an ice bath in the fridge for up to 2 days and reheat for serving.

Serving: Warm the poached egg in hot water for 30 seconds to 1 minute. Do not microwave as it will overcook the egg.

Toast the bread, spread fresh avocado, and place the reheated poached egg on top.

Shrimp & Zucchini Noodles

Preparation Time: 10 minutes
Cooking Time: 10 minutes
Servings: 1

Ingredients:
4 oz Shrimp, peeled and deveined
1 medium Zucchini, spiralized
1 tbsp Olive Oil
1 tbsp Lemon Juice
Salt and Pepper, to taste

Instructions: In a skillet, heat olive oil and cook shrimp until pink.
Add zucchini noodles and cook until tender.
Drizzle with lemon juice and season with salt and pepper.
Serve immediately.

Nutrient	Amount
Calories	250 kcal
Protein	25g
Total Carbohydrates	10g
- Sugars	5g
- Dietary Fiber	2g
Total Fat	15g
- Saturated Fat	2g

Meal Prepping:
Storage: Store in an airtight container in the refrigerator for up to 2 days.
Serving: Reheat gently in a skillet over medium heat for 2-3 minutes.

Turkey & Quinoa Stuffed Peppers

Preparation Time: 15 minutes

Cooking Time: 30 minutes

Servings: 1

Ingredients:

1 large Bell Pepper, halved and seeded

4 oz Ground Turkey

½ cup Cooked Quinoa

1 tbsp Olive Oil

Salt and Pepper, to taste

Instructions: Preheat oven to 375°F (190°C).

In a skillet, heat olive oil and cook turkey until browned.

Mix cooked turkey with quinoa and stuff into bell pepper halves.

Bake for 30 minutes or until peppers are tender.

Serve immediately.

Nutrient	Amount
Calories	350 kcal
Protein	30g
Total Carbohydrates	30g
- Sugars	5g
- Dietary Fiber	5g
Total Fat	15g
- Saturated Fat	3g

Meal Prepping:

Storage: Store in an airtight container in the refrigerator for up to 3-4 days.

Serving: Reheat in the microwave for 2-3 minutes or in a preheated oven at 350°F (175°C) for 10-15 minutes.

Egg & Spinach Scramble

Preparation Time: 5 minutes
Cooking Time: 5 minutes
Servings: 1

Ingredients:
3 large Eggs, whisked
1 cup Fresh Spinach
1 tbsp Olive Oil
Salt and Pepper, to taste

Instructions: In a skillet, heat olive oil and sauté spinach until wilted. Add whisked eggs and cook, stirring, until eggs are set. Season with salt and pepper. Serve immediately.

Nutrient	Amount
Calories	300 kcal
Protein	20g
Total Carbohydrates	5g
- Sugars	1g
- Dietary Fiber	1g
Total Fat	25g
- Saturated Fat	6g

Meal Prepping:
Storage: Store in an airtight container in the refrigerator for up to 1 day.
Serving: Reheat in the microwave for 1-1.5 minutes, stirring halfway through.

Protein Smoothie Bowl

Preparation Time: 5 minutes
Cooking Time: 0 minutes
Servings: 1

Ingredients:
1 scoop Protein Powder
1 cup Almond Milk
½ medium Banana, sliced
½ cup Mixed Berries
1 tbsp Almond Butter

Instructions: Blend protein powder, almond milk, and banana until smooth. Pour into a bowl and top with mixed berries and almond butter. Serve immediately.

Nutrient	Amount
Calories	350 kcal
Protein	30g
Total Carbohydrates	35g
- Sugars	20g
- Dietary Fiber	6g
Total Fat	15g
- Saturated Fat	2g

Meal Prepping:
Storage: Store in an airtight container in the refrigerator for up to 1 day. Note that consistency may change.
Serving: Serve chilled.

Veggie & Chicken Stir-Fry

Preparation Time: 10 minutes
Cooking Time: 15 minutes
Servings: 1

Ingredients:
4 oz Chicken Breast, sliced
1 cup Mixed Vegetables (bell peppers, snap peas, carrots), sliced
1 tbsp Soy Sauce
1 tbsp Olive Oil
1 tsp Sesame Seeds

Instructions: In a skillet, heat olive oil and cook chicken until browned. Add vegetables and soy sauce, and stir-fry until vegetables are tender. Sprinkle with sesame seeds and serve immediately.

Nutrient	Amount
Calories	350 kcal
Protein	30g
Total Carbohydrates	20g
- Sugars	5g
- Dietary Fiber	4g
Total Fat	15g
- Saturated Fat	2.5g

Meal Prepping:

Storage: Store the pancakes in an airtight container in the refrigerator for up to 3-4 days.

Serving: Reheat in a skillet over medium heat for 5 minutes or in the microwave for 2-3 minutes.

Cottage Cheese & Pineapple Bowl

Preparation Time: 5 minutes

Cooking Time: 0 minutes

Servings: 1

Ingredients:
1 cup Cottage Cheese
½ cup Pineapple Chunks
1 tbsp Honey
1 tbsp Walnuts, chopped

Instructions: In a bowl, mix cottage cheese and pineapple. Drizzle with honey and top with chopped walnuts. Serve immediately.

Nutrient	Amount
Calories	300 kcal
Protein	25g
Total Carbohydrates	35g
- Sugars	25g
- Dietary Fiber	2g
Total Fat	10g
- Saturated Fat	3g

Meal Prepping:

<u>Storage:</u> Store ingredients separately in the refrigerator for up to 2 days.

<u>Serving:</u> Mix cottage cheese and pineapple, drizzle with honey, and sprinkle with walnuts just before serving.

Almond & Berry Protein Shake

Preparation Time: 5 minutes

Cooking Time: 0 minutes

Servings: 1

Ingredients:

1 scoop Protein Powder

1 cup Almond Milk

½ cup Mixed Berries

1 tbsp Almond Butter

Instructions: Blend all ingredients until smooth. Serve immediately.

Nutrient	Amount
Calories	350 kcal
Protein	30g
Total Carbohydrates	25g
- Sugars	15g
- Dietary Fiber	5g
Total Fat	15g
- Saturated Fat	1g

Meal Prepping:

Storage: Store it in the refrigerator for up to 1 day.

Note that separation might occur.

Serving: Stir or shake well before serving. Serve chilled.

9 Vegetarian and Vegan Delights

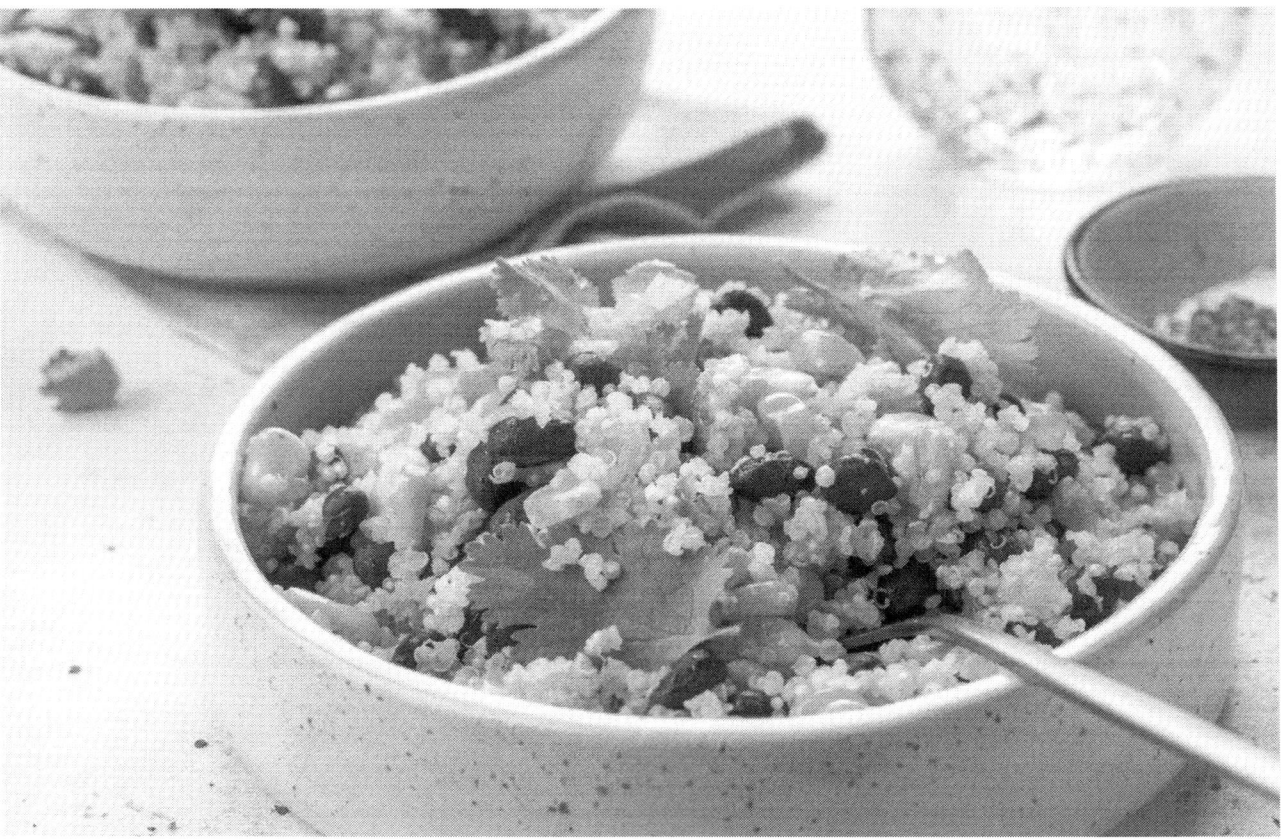

Quinoa & Black Bean Bowl - Page 122

Vegetarian and vegan recipes in bodybuilding meal prep require thoughtful planning to ensure that they meet the nutritional demands necessary for muscle growth and recovery, all while adhering to plant-based dietary restrictions. The primary challenge is obtaining sufficient protein, which is crucial for muscle repair and synthesis. Unlike omnivorous diets, plant-based regimens need a careful mix of protein sources to ensure a complete profile of essential amino acids.

Vegetarian and vegan bodybuilding recipes demand creativity and diversity in meal prep to maintain nutritional balance and prevent dietary boredom, all while supporting rigorous fitness goals.

Please note: the recipes are designed for one serving, allowing you the freedom to determine the number of meals you prepare in advance. Ensure you examine the food's condition before reheating and discard anything that appears or smells suspicious.

Vegan Chocolate Protein Shake

Preparation Time: 5 minutes
Cooking Time: 0 minutes
Servings: 1

Ingredients:
1 scoop Vegan Chocolate Protein Powder
1 cup Almond Milk
1 tbsp Almond Butter
1 tbsp Cocoa Powder

Instructions: Blend all ingredients until smooth. Serve immediately.

Nutrient	Amount
Calories	350 kcal
Protein	25g
Total Carbohydrates	25g
- Sugars	12g
- Dietary Fiber	4g
Total Fat	15g
- Saturated Fat	2g

Meal Prepping:

Storage: Store it in the refrigerator for up to 1 day.
Note that separation might occur.
Serving: Stir or shake well before serving. Serve chilled.

Vegan Protein Pancakes

Preparation Time: 10 minutes
Cooking Time: 10 minutes
Servings: 1

Ingredients:
1 scoop Vegan Protein Powder
½ cup Oat Flour
1 cup Almond Milk
1 tbsp Maple Syrup

Instructions: Mix protein powder, oat flour, and almond milk to form a batter. Cook pancakes on a griddle until golden on each side. Drizzle with maple syrup and serve immediately.

Nutrient	Amount
Calories	350 kcal
Protein	30g
Total Carbohydrates	40g
- Sugars	15g
- Dietary Fiber	4g
Total Fat	5g
- Saturated Fat	0.5g

Meal Prepping:

Storage: Store it in an airtight container in the refrigerator for up to 5 days or freeze for up to 2 months.

Serving: Reheat in the microwave for 20-30 seconds per pancake or in a toaster.

Vegan Protein Smoothie

Preparation Time: 5 minutes
Cooking Time: 0 minutes
Servings: 1

Ingredients:
1 scoop Vegan Protein Powder
1 cup Almond Milk
½ Banana
½ cup Mixed Berries

Instructions: Blend all ingredients until smooth. Serve immediately.

Nutrient	Amount
Calories	300 kcal
Protein	25g
Total Carbohydrates	40g
- Sugars	20g
- Dietary Fiber	6g
Total Fat	5g
- Saturated Fat	0.5g

Meal Prepping:

Storage: Store it in the refrigerator for up to 1 day.
Note that separation might occur.
Serving: Stir or shake well before serving. Serve chilled.

Vegetarian Omelette with Avocado & Tomato

Preparation Time: 10 minutes

Cooking Time: 10 minutes

Servings: 1

Ingredients:

3 large Eggs

½ Avocado, sliced

½ Tomato, sliced

1 tbsp Olive Oil

Salt and Pepper, to taste

Instructions: In a skillet, heat olive oil and pour whisked eggs. Add avocado and tomato slices and cook until eggs are set. Season with salt and pepper and serve immediately.

Nutrient	Amount
Calories	350 kcal
Protein	20g
Total Carbohydrates	15g
- Sugars	4g
- Dietary Fiber	5g
Total Fat	25g
- Saturated Fat	6g

Meal Prepping:

<u>Storage:</u> Store it in the refrigerator for up to 1 day.

<u>Serving:</u> Reheat in the microwave for 1-2 minutes or on a skillet over low heat.

Spicy Tofu & Vegetable Stir-Fry

Preparation Time: 10 minutes
Cooking Time: 15 minutes
Servings: 1

Ingredients:
4 oz Firm Tofu, cubed
1 cup Mixed Vegetables (bell peppers, snap peas, carrots), sliced
1 tbsp Soy Sauce
1 tbsp Olive Oil
1 tsp Sriracha Sauce

Instructions: In a skillet, heat olive oil and cook tofu until golden. Add vegetables, soy sauce, and Sriracha, and stir-fry until vegetables are tender. Serve immediately.

Nutrient	Amount
Calories	350 kcal
Protein	20g
Total Carbohydrates	30g
- Sugars	5g
- Dietary Fiber	5g
Total Fat	15g
- Saturated Fat	2g

Meal Prepping:

Storage: Store it in an airtight container in the refrigerator for up to 3-4 days.

Serving: Reheat in a skillet over medium heat for 5 minutes or in the microwave for 2-3 minutes.

Quinoa & Black Bean Bowl

Preparation Time: 10 minutes

Cooking Time: 20 minutes

Servings: 1

Ingredients:

½ cup Cooked Quinoa

½ cup Black Beans, cooked

½ cup Corn Kernels

1 tbsp Olive Oil

Salt and Pepper, to taste

Instructions: In a bowl, mix quinoa, black beans, and corn. Drizzle with olive oil and season with salt and pepper. Serve immediately.

Nutrient	Amount
Calories	350 kcal
Protein	15g
Total Carbohydrates	50g
- Sugars	2g
- Dietary Fiber	10g
Total Fat	10g
- Saturated Fat	1.5g

Meal Prepping:

Storage: Store it in an airtight container in the refrigerator for up to 5 days.

Serving: Reheat in the Microwave for 2-3 minutes, stirring halfway through, or warm in a skillet over medium heat.

Sweet Potato & Black Bean Burrito

Preparation Time: 15 minutes
Cooking Time: 20 minutes
Servings: 1

Ingredients:
1 medium Sweet Potato, diced
½ cup Black Beans, cooked
1 Whole Wheat Tortilla
1 tbsp Olive Oil
1 tbsp Salsa

Instructions: In a skillet, heat olive oil and cook sweet potato until tender. Mix sweet potato and black beans and wrap in a tortilla. Serve with salsa.

Nutrient	Amount
Calories	400 kcal
Protein	15g
Total Carbohydrates	60g
- Sugars	8g
- Dietary Fiber	10g
Total Fat	10g
- Saturated Fat	1.5g

Meal Prepping:

Storage: Wrap burritos tightly in foil and store in the refrigerator for up to 3 days or freeze for up to 1 month.

Serving: If refrigerated, microwave for 1-2 minutes. If frozen, thaw in the refrigerator overnight and microwave for 2-3 minutes, or heat in the oven at 350°F (175°C) for 10-15 minutes.

Vegetarian Greek Salad

Preparation Time: 10 minutes
Cooking Time: 0 minutes
Servings: 1

Ingredients:
1 cup Mixed Greens
½ cup Cherry Tomatoes, halved
½ cup Cucumber, sliced
¼ cup Feta Cheese, crumbled
1 tbsp Olive Oil
1 tbsp Balsamic Vinegar
Salt and Pepper, to taste

Instructions: In a bowl, mix greens, tomatoes, cucumber, and feta. Drizzle with olive oil and balsamic vinegar, and season with salt and pepper. Serve immediately.

Nutrient	Amount
Calories	250 kcal
Protein	10g
Total Carbohydrates	15g
- Sugars	5g
- Dietary Fiber	3g
Total Fat	15g
- Saturated Fat	5g

Meal Prepping:
Storage: Store ingredients separately in the refrigerator for up to 2 days.
Serving: Serve chilled or at room temperature. Drizzle dressing and toss just before serving.

Vegetarian Quiche with Spinach & Feta

Preparation Time: 15 minutes

Cooking Time: 30 minutes

Servings: 1

Ingredients:

3 large Eggs

1 cup Spinach, chopped

¼ cup Feta Cheese, crumbled

1 tbsp Olive Oil

Salt and Pepper, to taste

Instructions: In a skillet, heat olive oil and sauté spinach until wilted.

Pour whisked eggs over spinach and add feta.

Bake for 30 minutes or until set.

Season with salt and pepper and serve immediately.

Nutrient	Amount
Calories	350 kcal
Protein	20g
Total Carbohydrates	10g
- Sugars	2g
- Dietary Fiber	2g
Total Fat	25g
- Saturated Fat	8g

Meal Prepping:

Storage: Store in an airtight container in the refrigerator for up to 3 days.

Serving: Reheat in the oven at 350°F (175°C) for 10-15 minutes or in the microwave for 2-3 minutes.

Vegan Lentil & Vegetable Soup

Preparation Time: 15 minutes
Cooking Time: 30 minutes
Servings: 1

Ingredients:
½ cup Lentils, cooked
1 cup Mixed Vegetables (carrots, celery, potatoes), diced
2 cups Vegetable Broth
1 tbsp Olive Oil
Salt and Pepper, to taste

Instructions: In a pot, heat olive oil and sauté vegetables until golden. Add lentils and broth and simmer for 30 minutes. Season with salt and pepper and serve immediately.

Nutrient	Amount
Calories	350 kcal
Protein	20g
Total Carbohydrates	40g
- Sugars	6g
- Dietary Fiber	10g
Total Fat	10g
- Saturated Fat	1.5g

Meal Prepping:

<u>Storage:</u> Store in an airtight container in the refrigerator for up to 5 days or freeze for up to 2 months.

<u>Serving:</u> Reheat on the stovetop over medium heat or in the microwave for 3-4 minutes.

Vegetarian Cottage Cheese & Pineapple Bowl

Preparation Time: 10 minutes

Cooking Time: 0 minutes

Servings: 1

Ingredients:

1 cup Cottage Cheese

½ cup Pineapple, diced

1 tbsp Honey

1 tbsp Almonds, chopped

Instructions: In a bowl, mix cottage cheese, pineapple, honey, and almonds. Serve immediately.

Nutrient	Amount
Calories	300 kcal
Protein	25g
Total Carbohydrates	35g
- Sugars	25g
- Dietary Fiber	2g
Total Fat	10g
- Saturated Fat	4g

Meal Prepping:

Storage: Store it in an airtight container in the refrigerator for up to 1 day.

Serving: Serve chilled.

Vegetarian Protein Bars

Preparation Time: 15 minutes

Cooking Time: 20 minutes

Servings: 1

Ingredients:

1 scoop Vegetarian Protein Powder

½ cup Oat Flour

¼ cup Almond Butter

2 tbsp Honey

Instructions: Mix all ingredients and press into a baking dish. Bake for 20 minutes or until golden. Cool and cut into bars.

Nutrient	Amount
Calories	350 kcal
Protein	25g
Total Carbohydrates	35g
- Sugars	15g
- Dietary Fiber	4g
Total Fat	15g
- Saturated Fat	2.5g

Meal Prepping:

Storage: After chilling and cutting into bars, store them in an airtight container in the refrigerator for up to 7 days or freeze for up to 1 month.

Serving: These can be enjoyed cold or brought to room temperature for a softer texture.

10 Advanced Meal Prep Strategies

10.1 Batch Cooking and Freezing: A Lifesaver for the Busy Bodybuilder

Batch cooking and freezing transcend mere culinary convenience, emerging as strategic linchpins in the quest for nutritional excellence, particularly within the bodybuilding community. This dual approach not only ensures a consistent supply of nutritious meals, crucial for muscle repair and growth, but also serves as a testament to one's dedication to health and fitness goals. By delving into batch cooking, you're investing in a system designed to streamline your dietary efforts, mirroring the discipline and efficiency you apply to your workouts.

The essence of batch cooking lies in its capacity to prepare substantial food quantities, designed to sustain you over a period, thereby liberating your schedule from the constant need for cooking and redirecting that energy towards training and recovery. Freezing, the indispensable ally of batch cooking, locks in freshness and nutritional quality, ensuring each meal is a step towards your bodybuilding aspirations.

This approach safeguards the nutritional integrity of your diet, minimizing nutrient loss and giving your body the fundamental components it need. It also introduces an element of variety, warding off dietary monotony by offering a spectrum of flavors and nutrients essential for long-term diet adherence. Moreover, the time efficiency gained by dedicating a few hours to meal preparation each week is invaluable, freeing up hours for additional workouts, relaxation, or other personal endeavors. However, this system thrives on strategic planning, necessitating an organized approach to meal planning, shopping, and cooking, ultimately contributing to a well-rounded and diverse diet. Additionally, the economic prudence of batch cooking is undeniable, with bulk buying and reduced reliance on takeout leading to substantial savings, a boon considering the increased caloric intake often associated with bodybuilding. Finally, the discipline inherent in batch cooking — precise portion control — is crucial for those meticulously tracking their macronutrient intake, fortifying the commitment to their bodybuilding journey.

10.2 Optimizing Meal Timing: Synchronizing Nutrition with Your Body's Clock

Optimizing meal timing, an intricate facet of nutrition, holds the power to amplify the health and fitness journey by meticulously synchronizing food intake with the body's inherent rhythms and energy requisites, thereby enhancing metabolic function, fortifying fitness objectives, and nurturing an equilibrium with food. This journey of nutritional synchronization isn't solely about the substance of your meals but significantly about the timing, a strategic element that profoundly influences your health, vigor, and life's quality. Proper meal timing, a concept that transcends mere eating schedules, works in harmony with the body's metabolic cycles, energy demands, and workout routines, ensuring a constant supply of nutrients, bolstering energy levels, and supporting metabolic health.

For the devoted athlete or fitness aficionado, such timing is indispensable, providing the necessary fuel for enhanced performance and ensuring optimal recovery post-exercise. Moreover, the strategic timing of meals plays a crucial role in managing weight and honing body composition, with consistent meal intervals helping regulate appetite and optimize muscle growth and fat reduction. Aligning with the body's circadian rhythm, this approach not only supports physiological functions but also promotes overall well-being. It's a flexible, individualized strategy, demanding a tailored approach that accommodates one's unique lifestyle, preferences, and goals, promoting mindfulness and psychological satisfaction in eating habits.

Furthermore, emerging studies indicate potential long-term benefits, suggesting a link between synchronized meal timing and longevity, improved metabolic health, and a reduced risk of chronic conditions. Practical implementation involves meticulous planning, attentiveness to bodily cues, alignment with physical activity, and an emphasis on substantial breakfasts while avoiding late-night caloric intake, collectively fostering metabolic health and effective weight management.

11 Overcoming Challenges

11.1 Balancing Desires: Managing Cravings and Cheat Days

Managing cravings and cheat days involves a delicate balance of mindfulness, informed choices, and embracing culinary diversity, all while heeding your body's subtle signals and indulging with intention and restraint. Cravings, often the body's language for expressing needs, desires, or deficiencies, require discernment between emotional yearnings and physiological necessities, enabling more mindful, balanced food decisions. Introducing a variety of foods, flavors, and textures combats culinary monotony, satisfying your palate, diminishing cravings, and ensuring a comprehensive nutrient intake, making meals both exciting and nourishing.

Cheat days, though a tempting respite in a landscape of dietary discipline, demand mindful planning and moderation. Scheduled indulgences, focusing on quality and mindful savoring, can fulfill desires without nutritional derailment. Hydration is a critical ally in this journey, as the body can confuse thirst for hunger, prompting unwarranted snacking; consistent water consumption maintains equilibrium, curbs cravings, and bolsters overall health.

When cravings beckon, choosing healthier, nutrient-rich alternatives—like fruits or dark chocolate for sweets, or nuts for salty treats—aligns indulgence with nutritional objectives. Portion control acts as a navigational tool amidst culinary temptations, ensuring enjoyment without the aftermath of excess. Mindful eating, a practice of fully engaging the senses, enhances meal satisfaction, mitigating cravings and overeating.

Ultimately, commitment to one's nutritional and fitness aspirations is the anchor amidst the tempest of cravings. Recalling your foundational 'why' fortifies resolve, guiding you through cravings with steadfast determination, ensuring that each indulgence is a step not away from, but along the path to your health and wellness goals.

11.2 The Journey of Persistence: Staying Motivated and Consistent

Staying motivated and consistent in your bodybuilding meal prep journey harmonizes clear goals, a positive mindset, structured routine, communal support, continual learning, and celebrating progress into a symphony of growth and fulfillment. Clear, realistic goals act as your roadmap, providing direction and milestones that fuel your drive. A positive mindset, nurtured through affirmations, visualization, and gratitude, becomes your catalyst, empowering you to surmount challenges and learn from setbacks. Routine and structure breed consistency, morphing meal prep from daunting to seamless, while support from a community offers a wellspring of encouragement, advice, and accountability, making the journey less solitary and more purposeful.

Celebrating each small victory fosters a sense of progress, invigorating your commitment, while continuous education in nutrition and fitness acts as a compass, guiding your choices and keeping your motivation aflame. As your journey evolves, so should your goals; revisiting and refining them ensures they remain relevant, challenging, and inspiring, keeping your path purpose-driven. Ultimately, embracing the journey, with all its peaks and valleys, not only enriches your experience but also deepens your connection to your nutritional and fitness aspirations. This journey, punctuated by each small triumph and supported by knowledge and community, transforms from a mere routine into a dance of continual growth and fulfillment, each step a harmonious stride toward your ultimate vision of health and wellness.

11.3 Embarking on a Transformative Journey: Encouragement and Final Thoughts

As the curtain falls on this enlightening guide, a moment of reflection beckons, crystallizing the essence of the transformative journey of bodybuilding meal prep, a voyage not solely of the body but a holistic metamorphosis of mind and spirit, brimming with discovery, growth, and profound fulfillment. Embarking with an open heart and insatiable curiosity, this path unfolds as a boundless learning landscape, where each step, challenge, and moment blossoms into opportunities for deep self-discovery. The journey demands the nurturing of discipline and consistency, foundational pillars that, when watered with dedication and regularity, bloom into formidable strength and unwavering resilience, underscoring the journey's marathon nature, demanding patience and steadfast perseverance.

Central to this odyssey is the cultivation of a positive, empowering mindset, the architect crafting your transformative reality, turning challenges into stepping stones toward greater mastery. Life's symphony plays to the rhythm of balance and harmony, necessitating a delicate equilibrium among nutrition, exercise, rest, and personal life, composing a melody that resonates with holistic well-being. This journey weaves a rich tapestry of connection, sharing, and communal growth, fostering a supportive and enriching brotherhood of like-minded souls.

The true beauty of this expedition lies in cherishing the process and reveling in each triumph, no matter how small. As you poised at this journey's genesis, recognize it as a pilgrimage of self-discovery, mastery, and fulfillment, a harmonious dance intertwining physical nourishment with mental enrichment and spiritual efflorescence. So, with courage, passion, and unwavering self-belief, step forth; let this journey illuminate your path to transformation, empowerment, and the ultimate realization of your boundless potential, embodying the joy of continual growth and the actualization of your highest self.

12 Bonuses

12.1 My 30-Day Meal Plan

Meal planning, a cornerstone of clean eating, orchestrates a symphony of diverse, balanced diets, efficient time and resource management, and consistent healthy choices, transforming eating from a mundane task into a joyous journey toward health and happiness. This strategic approach, far from a mere schedule, serves as a nutritional compass, guiding adherents of clean eating through common hurdles like time constraints and monotony, thereby paving the way for a seamless transition to enduring healthy habits. It's not just about making clean eating manageable; it's about fostering a sustainable commitment to a nourishing lifestyle, a commitment that unfurls a tapestry of wellness benefits.

The crux of meal planning's importance lies in its capacity for efficiency, ensuring nutritional equilibrium, budget adherence, and steering clear of unhealthy pitfalls by having wholesome meals at the ready. The process, however, demands a methodical approach: evaluating nutritional needs and preferences, crafting a varied weekly menu, devising an organized grocery list, setting aside dedicated prep time, and calibrating portion sizes to match dietary needs. Clean eating accentuates whole, unprocessed foods, urging a rainbow of meal options and mindful portioning, all while allowing flexibility for life's unpredictability.

Moreover, practical strategies can ease the transition: beginning with manageable prep tasks, embracing batch cooking, investing in quality storage, planning diverse menus, utilizing time-saving gadgets, pre-portioning meals, labeling containers for clarity, and including freezer-friendly options. These tactics are not mere conveniences but vital steps in harmonizing one's lifestyle with the principles of clean eating, ensuring each meal is a stepping stone to a healthier existence.

This is my favorite 30-Day meal plan. Feel free to follow it verbatim or change the recipes to those I have included in the book, like vegetarian and vegan ones.

Day 1:
Breakfast: Protein-Packed Oatmeal
Lunch: Grilled Chicken & Quinoa Salad
Dinner: Baked Tilapia & Green Beans
Snack: Zucchini & Parmesan Chips
Post-Workout: Avocado & Egg Toast
Total Nutrients: Calories: 2050, Protein: 127g, Total Carbohydrates: 140g, Sugars: 30g, Dietary Fiber: 28g, Total Fat: 90g, Saturated Fat: 17.5g

Day 2:
Breakfast: Protein-Packed Oatmeal
Lunch: Grilled Chicken & Quinoa Salad
Dinner: Baked Tilapia & Green Beans
Snack: Zucchini & Parmesan Chips
Post-Workout: Avocado & Egg Toast
Total Nutrients: Calories: 2050, Protein: 127g, Total Carbohydrates: 140g, Sugars: 30g, Dietary Fiber: 28g, Total Fat: 90g, Saturated Fat: 17.5g

Day 3:
Breakfast: Protein-Packed Oatmeal
Lunch: Grilled Chicken & Quinoa Salad
Dinner: Beef Stir-Fry & Brown Rice
Snack: Power Protein Balls
Post-Workout: Almond & Berry Protein Shake
Total Nutrients: 2110 Calories, 160g Protein, 195g Total Carbohydrates, 51g Sugars, 26g Dietary Fiber, 90g Total Fat, 16g Saturated Fat

Day 4:
Breakfast: Protein-Packed Oatmeal
Lunch: Grilled Chicken & Quinoa Salad
Dinner: Beef Stir-Fry & Brown Rice
Snack: Power Protein Balls
Post-Workout: Shrimp & Zucchini Noodles
Total Nutrients: 2010 Calories, 160g Protein, 175g Total Carbohydrates, 39g Sugars, 23g Dietary Fiber, 85g Total Fat, 17g Saturated Fat

Day 5:
Breakfast: Almond Butter & Banana Smoothie
Lunch: Grilled Chicken & Quinoa Salad
Dinner: Beef Stir-Fry & Brown Rice
Snack: Nutty Protein Bars
Post-Workout: Shrimp & Zucchini Noodles
Total Nutrients: 1920 Calories, 165g Protein, 180g Total Carbohydrates, 44g Sugars, 28g Dietary Fiber, 87g Total Fat, 15g Saturated Fat

Day 6:
Breakfast: Egg White & Spinach Scramble
Lunch: Turkey & Veggie Lettuce Wraps
Dinner: Baked Cod & Asparagus
Snack: Nutty Protein Bars
Post-Workout: Protein Smoothie Bowl
Total Nutrients: 1570 Calories, 145g Protein, 160g Total Carbohydrates, 43g Sugars, 20g Dietary Fiber, 77g Total Fat, 15g Saturated Fat

Day 7:
Breakfast: Egg White & Spinach Scramble
Lunch: Turkey & Veggie Lettuce Wraps
Dinner: Baked Cod & Asparagus
Snack: Power Protein Balls
Post-Workout: Cottage Cheese & Pineapple Bowl
Total Nutrients: 1560 Calories, 145g Protein, 155g Total Carbohydrates, 48g Sugars, 19g Dietary Fiber, 67g Total Fat, 16g Saturated Fat

Day 8:
Breakfast: Egg White & Spinach Scramble
Lunch: Turkey & Veggie Lettuce Wraps
Dinner: Shrimp & Cauliflower Rice
Snack: Power Protein Balls
Post-Workout: Cottage Cheese & Pineapple Bowl
Total Nutrients: 1610 Calories, 145g Protein, 145g Total Carbohydrates, 48g Sugars, 19g Dietary Fiber, 87g Total Fat, 16g Saturated Fat

Day 9:
Breakfast: Protein Pancakes with Berry Compote
Lunch: Spicy Tuna Salad
Dinner: Shrimp & Cauliflower Rice
Snack: Protein-Packed Trail Mix
Post-Workout: Protein Pancakes
Total Nutrients: 1650 Calories, 133g Protein, 160g Total Carbohydrates, 52g Sugars, 28g Dietary Fiber, 83g Total Fat, 15g Saturated Fat

Day 10:
Breakfast: Protein Pancakes with Berry Compote
Lunch: Spicy Tuna Salad
Dinner: Turkey & Butternut Squash Hash
Snack: Protein-Packed Trail Mix
Post-Workout: Avocado & Egg Toast
Total Nutrients: 2050 Calories, 130g Protein, 190g Total Carbohydrates, 49g Sugars, 34g Dietary Fiber, 90g Total Fat, 18.5g Saturated Fat

Day 11:
Breakfast: Protein Pancakes with Berry Compote
Lunch: Spinach and Feta Stuffed Chicken
Dinner: Turkey & Butternut Squash Hash
Snack: Spicy Roasted Chickpeas
Post-Workout: Protein Pancakes
Total Nutrients: Calories: 1850, Protein: 140g, Total Carbohydrates: 170g, Sugars: 49g, Dietary Fiber: 28g, Total Fat: 76g, Saturated Fat: 18g

Day 12:
Breakfast: Protein Pancakes with Berry Compote
Lunch: Spinach and Feta Stuffed Chicken
Dinner: Turkey & Butternut Squash Hash
Snack: Spicy Roasted Chickpeas
Post-Workout: Salmon & Asparagus Bake
Total Nutrients: Calories: 1850, Protein: 135g, Total Carbohydrates: 140g, Sugars: 44g, Dietary Fiber: 26g, Total Fat: 86g, Saturated Fat: 19g

Day 13:
Breakfast: Veggie & Egg White Muffins
Lunch: Spinach and Feta Stuffed Chicken
Dinner: Vegetable & Quinoa Stuffed Peppers
Snack: Veggie Sticks with Hummus Dip
Post-Workout: Salmon & Asparagus Bake
Total Nutrients: Calories: 1430, Protein: 121g, Total Carbohydrates: 100g, Sugars: 19g, Dietary Fiber: 19g, Total Fat: 72g, Saturated Fat: 13g

Day 14:
Breakfast: Veggie & Egg White Muffins
Lunch: Spinach and Feta Stuffed Chicken
Dinner: Vegetable & Quinoa Stuffed Peppers
Snack: Veggie Sticks with Hummus Dip
Post-Workout: Mango & Cottage Cheese Bowl
Total Nutrients: Calories: 1430, Protein: 121g, Total Carbohydrates: 130g, Sugars: 47g, Dietary Fiber: 20g, Total Fat: 62g, Saturated Fat: 12.5g

Day 15:
Breakfast: Greek Yogurt & Nut Parfait
Lunch: Sweet Potato & Black Bean Bowl
Dinner: Vegetable & Quinoa Stuffed Peppers
Snack: Spicy Roasted Chickpeas
Post-Workout: Mango & Cottage Cheese Bowl
Total Nutrients: Calories: 1750, Protein: 100g, Total Carbohydrates: 225g, Sugars: 79g, Dietary Fiber: 35g, Total Fat: 60g, Saturated Fat: 12.5g

Day 16:
Breakfast: Greek Yogurt & Nut Parfait
Lunch: Sweet Potato & Black Bean Bowl
Dinner: Pork Chop with Green Beans and Almonds
Snack: Spicy Roasted Chickpeas
Post-Workout: Avocado & Egg Toast
Total Nutrients: Calories: 1950, Protein: 130g, Total Carbohydrates: 190g, Sugars: 53g, Dietary Fiber: 34g, Total Fat: 90g, Saturated Fat: 17.5g

Day 17:
Breakfast: Protein French Toast
Lunch: Sweet Potato & Black Bean Bowl
Dinner: Pork Chop with Green Beans and Almonds
Snack: Protein-Packed Trail Mix
Post-Workout: Avocado & Egg Toast
Total Nutrients: Calories: 2050, Protein: 133g, Total Carbohydrates: 190g, Sugars: 56g, Dietary Fiber: 30g, Total Fat: 100g, Saturated Fat: 20.5g

Day 18:
Breakfast: Sweet Potato & Turkey Sausage Hash
Lunch: Beef & Sweet Potato Hash
Dinner: Pork Chop with Green Beans and Almonds
Snack: Protein-Packed Trail Mix
Post-Workout: Protein Smoothie Bowl
Total Nutrients: Calories: 1950, Protein: 148g, Total Carbohydrates: 175g, Sugars: 49g, Dietary Fiber: 22g, Total Fat: 88g, Saturated Fat: 22.5g

Day 19:
Breakfast: Sweet Potato & Turkey Sausage Hash
Lunch: Beef & Sweet Potato Hash
Dinner: Shrimp and Broccoli Stir-Fry
Snack: Spicy Mixed Nuts
Post-Workout: Quinoa & Chicken Bowl
Total Nutrients: Calories: 1970, Protein: 145g, Total Carbohydrates: 145g, Sugars: 30g, Dietary Fiber: 20g, Total Fat: 115g, Saturated Fat: 20.5g

Day 20:
Breakfast: Sweet Potato & Turkey Sausage Hash
Lunch: Beef & Sweet Potato Hash
Dinner: Shrimp and Broccoli Stir-Fry
Snack: Spicy Mixed Nuts
Post-Workout: Quinoa & Chicken Bowl
Total Nutrients: Calories: 1970, Protein: 145g, Total Carbohydrates: 145g, Sugars: 30g, Dietary Fiber: 20g, Total Fat: 115g, Saturated Fat: 20.5g

Day 21:
Breakfast: Almond Butter & Banana Smoothie
Lunch: Shrimp & Veggie Salad
Dinner: Vegetable & Farro Stuffed Tomatoes
Snack: Spicy Mixed Nuts
Post-Workout: Quinoa & Chicken Bowl
Total Nutrients: Calories: 1850, Protein: 150g, Total Carbohydrates: 160g, Sugars: 74g, Dietary Fiber: 26g, Total Fat: 87g, Saturated Fat: 16.5g

Day 22:
Breakfast: Veggie & Egg Breakfast Burrito
Lunch: Shrimp & Veggie Salad
Dinner: Vegetable & Farro Stuffed Tomatoes
Snack: Berry & Oat Protein Bars
Post-Workout: Protein Pancakes
Total Nutrients: Calories: 1850, Protein: 145g, Total Carbohydrates: 170g, Sugars: 61g, Dietary Fiber: 30g, Total Fat: 75g, Saturated Fat: 13g

Day 23:
Breakfast: Veggie & Egg Breakfast Burrito
Lunch: Classic Grilled Chicken Quinoa Tabbouleh
Dinner: Vegetable & Farro Stuffed Tomatoes
Snack: Berry & Oat Protein Bars
Post-Workout: Protein Pancakes
Total Nutrients: Calories: 1900, Protein: 155g, Total Carbohydrates: 175g, Sugars: 62g, Dietary Fiber: 30g, Total Fat: 75g, Saturated Fat: 13g

Day 24:
Breakfast: Chia Seed & Berry Pudding
Lunch: Classic Grilled Chicken Quinoa Tabbouleh
Dinner: Chicken & Mango Salad
Snack: Berry & Oat Protein Bars
Post-Workout: Avocado & Egg Toast
Total Nutrients: Calories: 1750, Protein: 109g, Total Carbohydrates: 165g, Sugars: 59g, Dietary Fiber: 32g, Total Fat: 70g, Saturated Fat: 11.5g

Day 25:
Breakfast: Chia Seed & Berry Pudding
Lunch: Classic Grilled Chicken Quinoa Tabbouleh
Dinner: Chicken & Mango Salad
Snack: Nutty Protein Bars
Post-Workout: Avocado & Egg Toast
Total Nutrients: Calories: 1720, Protein: 127g, Total Carbohydrates: 155g, Sugars: 59g, Dietary Fiber: 26g, Total Fat: 80g, Saturated Fat: 12.5g

Day 26:
Breakfast: Chia Seed & Berry Pudding
Lunch: Classic Grilled Chicken Quinoa Tabbouleh
Dinner: Chicken & Mango Salad
Snack: Nutty Protein Bars
Post-Workout: Beef & Broccoli Stir-Fry
Total Nutrients: Calories: 1670, Protein: 147g, Total Carbohydrates: 135g, Sugars: 57g, Dietary Fiber: 25g, Total Fat: 90g, Saturated Fat: 14.5g

Day 27:
Breakfast: Chia Seed & Berry Pudding
Lunch: Salmon & Veggie Skewers
Dinner: Baked Cod & Asparagus
Snack: Zucchini & Parmesan Chips
Post-Workout: Beef & Broccoli Stir-Fry
Total Nutrients: Calories: 1550, Protein: 137g, Total Carbohydrates: 120g, Sugars: 52g, Dietary Fiber: 22g, Total Fat: 85g, Saturated Fat: 14.5g

Day 28:
Breakfast: Protein Pancakes with Berry Compote
Lunch: Salmon & Veggie Skewers
Dinner: Baked Cod & Asparagus
Snack: Zucchini & Parmesan Chips
Post-Workout: Beef & Broccoli Stir-Fry
Total Nutrients: Calories: 1750, Protein: 160g, Total Carbohydrates: 150g, Sugars: 72g, Dietary Fiber: 26g, Total Fat: 85g, Saturated Fat: 16.5g

Day 29:
Breakfast: Protein French Toast
Lunch: Spiced Lentil and Chicken Soup
Dinner: Spaghetti Squash & Turkey Meatballs
Snack: Spicy Roasted Chickpeas
Post-Workout: Chicken & Avocado Salad
Total Nutrients: Calories: 1900, Protein: 175g, Total Carbohydrates: 170g, Sugars: 64g, Dietary Fiber: 30g, Total Fat: 90g, Saturated Fat: 15.5g

Day 30:
Breakfast: Mango & Greek Yogurt Smoothie
Lunch: Spiced Lentil and Chicken Soup
Dinner: Spaghetti Squash & Turkey Meatballs
Snack: Spicy Roasted Chickpeas
Post-Workout: Chicken & Avocado Salad
Total Nutrients: Calories: 1800, Protein: 180g, Total Carbohydrates: 170g, Sugars: 65g, Dietary Fiber: 32g, Total Fat: 75g, Saturated Fat: 11.5g

12.2 Smart Grocery Shopping Tactics

In the realm of professional bodybuilding, meticulous dietary planning is paramount, optimizing muscle hypertrophy, recuperation, and holistic health. A glimpse into a pro bodybuilder's shopping list reveals a strategic nutritional blueprint, meticulously aligning food selections with the rigorous demands of their training and physique aspirations. Protein, the cornerstone of muscle synthesis, dominates the list, encompassing lean poultry, meats, comprehensive amino acid sources like eggs, omega-3-rich fish, and diverse plant-based options. Carbohydrates, the body's energy currency, are carefully chosen for their complexity and sustained release properties, with staples like sweet potatoes, whole grains, and an array of micronutrient-rich fruits and vegetables.

Not to be overshadowed, healthy fats, critical for hormonal equilibrium and muscle-building processes, find their way into the cart in the form of avocados, assorted nuts, seeds, and heart-healthy oils. The dairy aisle offers protein-packed Greek yogurt and cottage cheese, celebrated for their gut-friendly probiotics, alongside versatile low-calorie milk alternatives. While whole foods are the diet's bedrock, strategic supplementation with products like whey protein, BCAAs, and multivitamins ensures nutritional gaps are seamlessly bridged during grueling training spells. Hydration, too, is critical, with a preference for electrolyte-balanced options post-exertion and metabolism-boosting beverages like green tea and coffee.

Snacking isn't omitted but is instead a calculated maneuver involving nutrient-dense options to sustain energy and satiate appetite, ensuring unwavering adherence to their dietary regimen. The list concludes with an array of culinary enhancers — spices, herbs, and low-calorie condiments — infusing meals with flavorful diversity sans caloric surplus. This holistic, strategic alimentary compendium is not merely a shopping list but a testament to the symbiotic relationship between nutrition and bodybuilding, underscoring the imperative of informed, goal-aligned food choices in sculpting athletic success.

12.3 Colton Jones Sample Weekly Grocery list

Proteins:

Chicken (various cuts) - estimate 6-8 breasts for multiple recipes

Turkey (ground) - around 4 lbs for different dishes

Beef (ground, stir-fry cuts) - 3-4 lbs

Salmon - 4 fillets

Shrimp - 2 lbs

Tuna (canned) - 4 cans

Cod - 2 fillets

Tilapia - 2 fillets

Haddock - 2 fillets

Pork chops - 4 chops

Eggs - 2 dozen (considering uses in multiple recipes)

Greek yogurt - 2 large containers

Cottage cheese - 1 large container

Almond butter - 1 jar

Tofu - 2 blocks

Chickpeas - 4 cans or bags

Lentils - 1 bag

Quinoa - 2 bags

Protein powder - 1 container

Various nuts (almonds, walnuts, etc.) - 1 bag each

Vegetables/Fruits:

Spinach - 2 large bags

Berries (mixed) - 3 lbs

Mango - 4

Apple - 6

Banana - 1 bunch

Sweet potatoes - 8

Asparagus - 2 bunches

Broccoli - 2 heads or bags

Green beans - 2 lbs

Brussels sprouts - 1 lb

Zucchini - 6

Cauliflower - 2 heads

Peppers - 6

Tomatoes - 8

Avocado - 6

Pineapple - 2

Cabbage - 2 heads

Lettuce - 2 heads or bags

Squash varieties - 4 each type

Eggplant - 2

Carrots - 1 bag

Celery - 1 bunch

Grains/Seeds:

Oats - 2 large containers

Bulgur - 1 bag

Farro - 1 bag

Chia seeds - 1 bag

Rice varieties - 2 bags each

Pasta - 2 boxes

Bread (whole grain) - 2 loaves

Dairy/Non-Dairy:

Milk (varieties) - 2 gallons

Cheese varieties - 1 block or bag each

Butter - 1 lb

Herbs/Spices/Condiments:

Cinnamon - 1 container

Various fresh herbs - small bunches

Spices (assorted) - 1 container each

Salsa - 1 jar

Soy sauce - 1 bottle

Hot sauce - 1 bottle

Olive oil - 1 bottle

Vinegars - 1 bottle each

Honey - 1 bottle

Snacks:

Trail mix ingredients - according to preference

Beverages:

Tea/Coffee - as needed

Almond milk (for shakes) - 1 gallon

13 Alphabetical Recipe Index

A

Almond & Berry Protein Shake - Page 115

Almond Butter & Banana Smoothie - Page 25

Apple & Cinnamon Oatmeal - Page 33

Avocado & Egg Toast - Page 108

B

Baked Cod & Asparagus - Page 65

Baked Haddock & Roasted Vegetables - Page 84

Baked Salmon & Steamed Veggies - Page 62

Baked Sweet Potato Fries - Page 92

Baked Tilapia & Green Beans - Page 77

Beef & Broccoli Stir-Fry - Page 105

Beef & Brussels Sprouts Stir-Fry - Page 79

Beef & Cabbage Stir-Fry - Page 86

Beef & Sweet Potato Hash - Page 45

Beef & Veggie Bowl - Page 54

Beef & Veggie Stir-Fry - Page 49

Berry & Oat Protein Bars - Page 95

C

Chicken & Avocado Salad - Page 103

Chicken & Mango Salad - Page 78

Chicken & Pineapple Salad - Page 85

Chicken & Pumpkin Curry - Page 81

Chicken & Sweet Potato Curry - Page 73

Chicken & Veggie Kabobs - Page 53

Chicken & Veggie Pasta - Page 48

Chicken & Veggie Skewers - Page 60

Chicken & Vegetable Curry - Page 66

Chickpea and Quinoa Salad - Page 50

Chia Seed & Berry Pudding - Page 28

Classic Grilled Chicken Quinoa Tabbouleh - Page 52

Classic Grilled Chicken Salad - Page 39

Cottage Cheese & Pineapple Bowl - Page 114

E

Egg & Spinach Scramble - Page 111

Egg White & Spinach Scramble - Page 21

G

Greek Yogurt & Nut Parfait - Page 23

Grilled Chicken & Quinoa Salad - Page 36

M

Mango & Cottage Cheese Bowl - Page 106

Mango & Greek Yogurt Smoothie - Page 31

N

Nutty Protein Bars - Page 90

O

Oatmeal & Berry Bowl - Page 107

P

Pesto Grilled Shrimp Quinoa Bowl - Page 55

Pork Chop with Green Beans and Almonds - Page 70

Power Protein Balls - Page 88

Protein French Toast - Page 29

Protein Pancakes - Page 104

Protein Pancakes with Berry Compote - Page 27

Protein Smoothie Bowl - Page 112

Protein-Packed Muesli - Page 34

Protein-Packed Oatmeal - Page 20

Protein-Packed Trail Mix - Page 93

Q
Quinoa & Berry Breakfast Bowl - Page 30

Quinoa & Black Bean Bowl - Page 122

Quinoa & Chicken Bowl - Page 100

Quinoa & Egg Breakfast Bowl - Page 22

Quinoa & Vegetable Salad - Page 89

S
Salmon & Asparagus Bake - Page 102

Salmon & Veggie Pasta - Page 59

Salmon & Veggie Skewers - Page 47

Salmon with Asparagus and Brown Rice - Page 68

Shrimp & Cauliflower Rice - Page 74

Shrimp & Veggie Salad - Page 51

Shrimp & Veggie Stir-Fry - Page 57

Shrimp & Zucchini Noodles - Page 109

Spaghetti Squash & Chicken Parmesan - Page 72

Spaghetti Squash & Turkey Meatballs - Page 64

Spiced Lentil and Chicken Soup - Page 41

Spicy Chicken & Rice Bowl - Page 44

Spicy Mixed Nuts - Page 94

Spicy Roasted Chickpeas - Page 91

Spicy Tofu & Vegetable Stir-Fry - Page 121

Spicy Tuna & Veggie Wrap - Page 56

Spicy Tuna Salad - Page 38

Spinach and Feta Stuffed Chicken - Page 43

Sweet Potato & Black Bean Bowl – Page 40

Sweet Potato & Black Bean Burrito - Page 123

Sweet Potato & Turkey Sausage Hash - Page 24

Sweet Potato & Turkey Skillet - Page 101

T
Turkey & Acorn Squash Hash - Page 82

Turkey & Butternut Squash Hash - Page 75

Turkey & Quinoa Stuffed Peppers - Page 110

Turkey & Sweet Potato Hash - Page 67

Turkey & Veggie Bowl - Page 58

Turkey & Veggie Lettuce Wraps - Page 46

Turkey & Veggie Skillet - Page 37

V
Vegan Chocolate Protein Shake - Page 117

Vegan Lentil & Vegetable Soup - Page 126

Vegan Protein Pancakes - Page 118

Vegan Protein Smoothie - Page 119

Vegetable & Bulgur Stuffed Eggplant - Page 83

Vegetable & Egg Fried Rice - Page 80

Vegetable & Farro Stuffed Tomatoes - Page 76

Vegetable & Quinoa Stuffed Peppers - Page 69

Veggie & Chicken Stir-Fry - Page 113

Veggie & Egg Breakfast Burrito - Page 32

Veggie & Egg White Muffins - Page 26

Veggie & Quinoa Bites - Page 96

Veggie & Quinoa Stir-Fry - Page 42

Veggie Sticks with Hummus Dip - Page 97

Z
Zucchini & Parmesan Chips - Page 98

Made in United States
Orlando, FL
09 December 2023